theclinics.com

PEDIATRIC CLINICS
OF NORTH AMERICA

Language, Communication, and Literacy: Pathologies and Treatments

GUEST EDITORS
Robert L. Russell, PhD
Mark D. Simms, MD, MPH

June 2007 • Volume 54 • Number 3

SAUNDERS

An Imprint of Elsevier, Inc.
PHILADELPHIA   LONDON   TORONTO   MONTREAL   SYDNEY   TOKYO

W.B. SAUNDERS COMPANY
A Division of Elsevier Inc.

1600 John F. Kennedy Boulevard • Suite 1800 • Philadelphia, Pennsylvania 19103

http://www.theclinics.com

THE PEDIATRIC CLINICS OF NORTH AMERICA
June 2007
Editor: Carla Holloway

Volume 54, Number 3
ISSN 0031-3955
ISBN-13: 978-1-4160-4354-6
ISBN-10: 1-4160-4354-3

The ideas and opinions expressed in *The Pediatric Clinics of North America* do not necessarily reflect those of the Publisher. The Publisher does not assume any responsibility for any injury and/or damage to persons or property arising out of or related to any use of the material contained in this periodical. The reader is advised to check the appropriate medical literature and the product information currently provided by the manufacturer of each drug to be administered to verify the dosage, the method and duration of administration, or contraindications. It is the responsibility of the treating physician or other health care professional, relying on independent experience and knowledge of the patient, to determine drug dosages and the best treatment for the patient. Mention of any product in this issue should not be construed as endorsement by the contributors, editors, or the Publisher of the product or manufacturers' claims.

The Pediatric Clinics of North America (ISSN 0031-3955) is published bi-monthly by Elsevier Inc. 360 Park Avenue South, New York, NY 10010-1710. Months of publication are February, April, June, August, October, and December. Business and Editorial Offices: 1600 John F. Kennedy Blvd., Suite 1800, Philadelphia, PA 19103-2899. Customer Service Office: 6277 Sea Harbor Drive, Orlando, FL 32887-4800. Periodicals postage paid at New York, NY and additional mailing offices. Subscription prices are $138.00 per year (US individuals), $281.00 per year (US institutions), $187.00 per year (Canadian individuals), $367.00 per year (Canadian institutions), $209.00 per year (international individuals), $367.00 per year (international institutions), $72.00 per year (US students), $110.00 per year (Canadian students), and $110.00 per year (foreign students). To receive students/resident rare, orders must be accompanied by name of affiliated institution, date of term, and the signature of program/residency coordinator on institution letterhead. Orders will be billed at individual rate until proof of status is received. Foreign air speed delivery is included in all Clinics subscription prices. All prices are subject to change without notice. POSTMASTER: Send address changes to *The Pediatric Clinics of North America*, Elsevier Periodicals Customer Service, 6277 Sea Harbor Drive, Orlando, FL 32887-4800. **Customer Service: 1-800-654-2452 (US). From outside of the US, call 1-407-345-4000**. E-mail: hhspcs@harcourt.com.

The Pediatric Clinics of North America is also published in Spanish by McGraw-Hill Inter-americana Editores S.A., Mexico City, Mexico; in Portuguese by Riechmann and Affonso Editores, Rua Comandante Coelho 1085, CEP 21250, Rio de Janeiro, Brazil; and in Greek by Althayia SA, Athens, Greece.

The Pediatric Clinics of North America is covered in *Index Medicus, Excerpta Medica, Current Contents, Current Contents/Clinical Medicine, Science Citation Index, ASCA, ISI/BIOMED*, and *BIOSIS*.

Printed in the United States of America.

GUEST EDITORS

ROBERT L. RUSSELL, PhD, Professor of Pediatrics, Medical College of Wisconsin; and Director of Research, Child Development Center, Children's Hospital of Wisconsin, Milwaukee, Wisconsin

MARK D. SIMMS, MD, MPH, Professor and Chief, Section of Developmental Pediatrics, Department of Pediatrics, Medical College of Wisconsin; and Child Development Center, Children's Hospital of Wisconsin, Milwaukee, Wisconsin

CONTRIBUTORS

ELIZABETH CARONNA, MD, Assistant Professor of Pediatrics, Division of Developmental and Behavioral Pediatrics, Boston Medical Center, Boston, Massachusetts

NANCY J. COHEN, PhD, Professor of Psychiatry and Director of Research, Hincks-Dellcrest Institute, Department of Psychiatry, University of Toronto, Toronto, Ontario, Canada

HEIDI M. FELDMAN, MD, PhD, Ballinger-Swindells Endowed Professor of Developmental and Behavioral Pediatrics, Department of Pediatrics, Stanford University School of Medicine, Palo Alto, California

KENNETH L. GRIZZLE, PhD, Assistant Professor, Department of Pediatrics, Medical College of Wisconsin, Children's Hospital of Wisconsin, Wauwatosa, Wisconsin

JEFFREY R. GRUEN, MD, Associate Professor of Pediatrics, Department of Pediatrics, Division of Neonatology, Yale University School of Medicine, New Haven, Connecticut

MARTHA R. HERBERT, MD, PhD, Assistant Professor, Department of Neurology, Massachusetts General Hospital, MGH/Martinos, Charlestown; and TRANSCEND Research Program, Center for Child and Adolescent Development, Cambridge Health Alliance, Harvard Medical School, Medford, Massachusetts

NANCIE IM-BOLTER, PhD, Assistant Professor of Psychology, Department of Psychology, Otonabee College, Trent University, Peterborough, Ontario, Canada

CLAUDIA KABLER-BABBITT, Program Coordinator, Department of Pediatrics, Medical College of Wisconsin, Milwaukee, Wisconsin

TAL KENET, PhD, Instructor, Harvard Medical School, Department of Neurology, Massachusetts General Hospital, MGH/Martinos, Charlestown, Massachusetts

LAUREN M. McGRATH, MA, Doctoral Candidate, Department of Psychology, University of Denver, Denver, Colorado

BRUCE F. PENNINGTON, PhD, John Evans Professor of Psychology, Department of Psychology; and Director, Developmental Neuropsychology Laboratory, University of Denver, Colorado

ROBIN L. PETERSON, MA, Doctoral Candidate, Department of Psychology, University of Denver, Denver, Colorado

ROBERT L. RUSSELL, PhD, Professor of Pediatrics, Medical College of Wisconsin; and Director of Research, Child Development Center, Children's Hospital of Wisconsin, Milwaukee, Wisconsin

ROBERT L. SCHUM, PhD, Associate Professor of Pediatrics, Section of Child Development, Department of Pediatrics, Medical College of Wisconsin; and Clinical Psychologist, Child Development Center, Children's Hospital of Wisconsin, Milwaukee, Wisconsin

BENNETT A. SHAYWITZ, MD, Professor of Pediatrics and Neurology, and Chief, Department of Pediatrics, Division of Child Neurology; and Co-Director, Yale Center for the Study of Learning, Reading, and Attention, Yale University School of Medicine, New Haven, Connecticut

SALLY E. SHAYWITZ, MD, Professor of Pediatrics, Department of Pediatrics, Division of Child Neurology; and Co-Director, Yale Center for the Study of Learning, Reading, and Attention, Yale University School of Medicine, New Haven, Connecticut

MARK D. SIMMS, MD, MPH, Professor and Chief, Section of Developmental Pediatrics, Department of Pediatrics, Medical College of Wisconsin; and Child Development Center, Children's Hospital of Wisconsin, Milwaukee, Wisconsin

SHELLEY D. SMITH, PhD, Professor of Pediatrics, Department of Pediatrics; and Chief, Hattie B. Munroe Molecular Genetics, University of Nebraska Medical Center, Omaha, Nebraska

HELEN TAGER-FLUSBERG, PhD, Professor, Department of Anatomy and Neurobiology, Boston University School of Medicine, Boston, Massachusetts

EARNESTINE WILLIS, MD, MPH, Associate Professor, Department of Pediatrics, Medical College of Wisconsin, Milwaukee, Wisconsin

BARRY ZUCKERMAN, MD, Chair and Professor, Department of Pediatrics, Boston City Hospital, Boston, Massachusetts

CONTENTS

PEDIATRIC CLINICS OF NORTH AMERICA JUNE 2007

GOAL STATEMENT

The goal of the *Pediatric Clinics of North America* is to keep practicing physicians and residents up to date with current clinical practice in pediatrics by providing timely articles reviewing the state-of-the-art in patient care.

ACCREDITATION

The *Pediatric Clinics of North America* is planned and implemented in accordance with the Essential Areas and Policies of the Accreditation Council for Continuing Medical Education (ACCME) through the joint sponsorship of the University Of Virginia School Of Medicine and Elsevier. The University Of Virginia School of Medicine is accredited by the ACCME to provide continuing medical education for physicians.

The University of Virginia School of Medicine designates this educational activity for a maximum of 15 *AMA PRA Category 1 Credits*™. Physicians should only claim credit commensurate with the extent of their participation in the activity.

The American Medical Association has determined that physicians not licensed in the US who participate in this CME activity are eligible for 15 *AMA PRA Category 1 Credits*™.

Credit can be earned by reading the text material, taking the CME examination online at http://www.theclinics.com/home/cme, and completing the evaluation. After taking the test, you will be required to review any and all incorrect answers. Following completion of the test and evaluation, your credit will be awarded and you may print your certificate.

FACULTY DISCLOSURE/CONFLICT OF INTEREST

The University of Virginia School of Medicine, as an ACCME accredited provider, endorses and strives to comply with the Accreditation Council for Continuing Medical Education (ACCME) Standards of Commercial Support, Commonwealth of Virginia statutes, University of Virginia policies and procedures, and associated federal and private regulations and guidelines on the need for disclosure and monitoring of proprietary and financial interests that may affect the scientific integrity and balance of content delivered in continuing medical education activities under our auspices.

The University of Virginia School of Medicine requires that all CME activities accredited through this institution be developed independently and be scientifically rigorous, balanced and objective in the presentation/discussion of its content, theories and practices.

All authors/editors participating in an accredited CME activity are expected to disclose to the readers relevant financial relationships with commercial entities occurring within the past 12 months (such as grants or research support, employee, consultant, stock holder, member of speakers bureau, etc.). The University of Virginia School of Medicine will employ appropriate mechanisms to resolve potential conflicts of interest to maintain the standards of fair and balanced education to the reader. Questions about specific strategies can be directed to the Office of Continuing Medical Education, University of Virginia School of Medicine, Charlottesville, Virginia.

The authors/editors listed below have identified no financial or professional relationships for themselves or their spouse/partner:
Elizabeth Caronna, MD; Nancy J. Cohen, PhD; Heidi M. Feldman, MD, PhD; Kenneth L. Grizzle, PhD; Jeffrey R. Gruen, MD; Martha R. Herbert, MD, PhD; Carla Holloway (Acquisitions Editor); Nancie Im-Bolter, PhD; Claudia Kabler-Babbitt, BSA; Tal Kenet, PhD; Lauren M. McGrath, MA; Bruce F. Pennington, PhD; Robin L. Peterson, MA; Robert L. Russell, PhD (Guest Editor); Robert L. Schum, PhD; Bennett A. Shaywitz, MD; Sally Shaywitz, MD; Mark D. Simms, MD, MPH; Shelley D. Smith, PhD; Helen Tager-Flusberg, PhD; and, Earnestine Willis, MD, MPH.

The authors/editors listed below identified the following professional or financial affiliations for themselves or their spouse/partner:
Barry Zuckerman, MD is a consultant for Reach Out and Read.

Disclosure of Discussion of Non-FDA Approved Uses for Pharmaceutical and/or Medical Device:
The University of Virginia School of Medicine, as an ACCME provider, requires that all authors identify and disclose any "off label" uses for pharmaceutical and medical device products. The University of Virginia School of Medicine recommends that each physician fully review all the available data on new products or procedures prior to clinical use.

TO ENROLL

To enroll in the *Pediatric Clinics of North America* Continuing Medical Education program, call customer service at 1-800-654-2452 or visit us online at *www.theclinics.com/home/cme*. The CME program is available to subscribers for an additional fee of $195.00

FORTHCOMING ISSUES

RECENT ISSUES

Preface

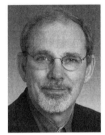 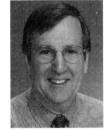

Robert L. Russell, PhD   Mark D. Simms, MD, MPH
Guest Editors

Roughly 69% of children served by the Individuals with Disabilities Education Act have either a specific learning disability (50%), which includes disorders of the basic processes involved in the use of spoken or written language, or speech or language impairment. These disorders can include dyslexia, spelling, and writing disorders; speech and language disorders; stuttering; and disorders with language impairment as one of the defining symptoms, such as in autism. Roughly about 4,257,000 children are expected to receive special education services for these disabilities, at a cost of over $33 billion [1,2]. The rate of comorbid psychiatric illness and psychosocial problems in children with developmental speech or language disabilities ranges between 20% and 50%. Both the *Diagnostic and Statistical Manual-IV* and the International Statistical Classification of Diseases and Related Health Problems-10 recognize the high rates of comorbidity, albeit to different degrees. In the United States, this means that roughly 851,000 to 2,128,500 children can be expected to need psychiatric or psychologic services, adding billions of more dollars to the societal economic burden, not to mention the increased suffering of the affected children and their families. These figures do not take into account that children with speech and language disorders are at increased risk of being victims of bullying, suffer social ostracism, and often feel alone.

Importantly, language learning delays and specific language and speech impairments can be identified early in childhood, and severe impairments can be indicative of a host of neurodevelopmental, genetic, autistic spectrum, or brain disorders with and without mental retardation. The pediatrician or family practitioner is the health care provider who is likely to have the first opportunity to observe and identify emerging language, communication, and

0031-3955/07/$ - see front matter © 2007 Elsevier Inc. All rights reserved.
doi:10.1016/j.pcl.2007.03.001

literacy problems and seek appropriate interventions. Impairments in aspects of language and communication are the most common disorders seen in healthy children in the years before and including kindergarten. Because of the many implications these disorders can have for the child's current and later overall functioning, pediatricians and family practitioners need to be able to recognize speech and language disorders when they occur and to understand available therapies to advise parents seeking help for their child. Moreover, with the increased attention to problems of autism and Asperger's syndrome, early detection of deficits in language and social responsivity has become crucial. As professionals, pediatricians and family practitioners should also be aware of the gains made in the understanding of the biologic bases of these disorders, because knowledge in genetics and neurosciences has grown considerably over the past decade.

For these reasons, it is important for pediatricians and family practitioners, along with their medical support staff, to acquaint themselves with the research and clinical literature focused on developmental language, communication, and literacy delays and disorders and how they impact important areas of cognitive and socioemotional functioning. This issue of the *Pediatric Clinics of North America* is designed to provide critical information on language, communication, and literacy impairments and their treatment, with information on how problems in these areas link to medical, brain, genetic, and psychiatric abnormalities. Articles are provided to guide practitioners through practicable screening diagnostics that can be used in the office, and what treatments are currently available. Moreover, given rapid developments in the genetics and neurobiology of these disorders, summaries of what is known about these areas are also provided. This issue is not meant to be a compendium or to provide practice guidelines. The experts included in this issue, however, have provided a well-rounded primer in a set of childhood disorders whose high incidence and prevalence rates guarantee that the pediatrician and family practitioner often are confronted with them in his or her office.

Robert L. Russell, PhD
Medical College of Wisconsin
8701 Watertown Plank Road
PO Box 26509, Milwaukee, WI 53226, USA

E-mail address: rrussell@mcw.edu

Mark D. Simms, MD, MPH
Child Development Center
Children's Hospital of Wisconsin
8701 Watertown Plank Road
PO Box 26509
Milwaukee, WI 53226, USA

E-mail address: msimms@mcw.edu

References

[1] Special Education-IDEA. IDEA funding coalition offers proposal. Washington DC: National Education Association; 2002.

[2] To assure the free appropriate public education of all children with disabilities. Twenty-fourth Annual Report to Congress on the Implementation of the Individuals with Disabilities Act. U.S. Department of Education, Office of Special Education Programs; 2002.

ELSEVIER
SAUNDERS

PEDIATRIC CLINICS
OF NORTH AMERICA

Pediatr Clin N Am 54 (2007) xv

Erratum

In the April 2007 issue of *Pediatric Clinics of North America* (Volume 54, Issue 2), an error appears in the article "Protecting Children from Toxic Exposure: Three Strategies" by Tee L. Guidotti and Lisa Ragain. The word "high" should be substituted for the word "low" on page 231, third full paragraph, sentence two. The sentence should read, "Most experts, however, now believe that this level of concern is too high because evidence for neurodevelopmental effects, in the form of group differences in IQ and academic achievement and a higher probability of behavioral abnormalities (including aggression), have been demonstrated even below this level [20–24]."

doi:10.1016/j.pcl.2007.05.001

Language Screening in the Pediatric Office Setting

Robert L. Schum, PhD[a,b,]*

[a]*Section of Child Development, Department of Pediatrics, Medical College of Wisconsin,
8701 Watertown Plank Road, Milwaukee, WI 53226, USA*
[b]*Child Development Center, Children's Hospital of Wisconsin,
P.O. Box 1997—MS #744, Milwaukee, WI 53201, USA*

Speech and language are core skills in the development of young children. They are markers of cognitive and social development, and also indicate certain features of motor development. Pediatricians routinely evaluate speech and language in well-child visits during the toddler and preschool years, as part of the developmental screening recommended by the American Academy of Pediatrics and the Center for Disease Control and Prevention [1]. Studies have indicated that speech and language delays occur at prevalence rates of 2% to 19%, depending upon how they are defined [2]. The purpose of this article is to discuss screening for language problems in a pediatric office setting.

Language and speech are distinguished for professional purposes. Speech refers to the production of sounds for the communication act. Language typically refers to four domains, each with a distinctive role. Language includes the rules that assign meaning to words and strings of words (semantics), the rules for combining words into phrases and sentences (syntax), the rules for combining the sounds of language (phonology), and the rules for the social use of language (pragmatics). Language skills include both reception and expression; that is, the child has an ability to understand an incoming message, and formulate and express an outgoing message. Language is commonly thought of in its spoken form, but it can also include a visual form, such as American Sign Language, which has all the key components of language, including a grammar system.

* Child Development Center, Children's Hospital of Wisconsin, P.O. Box 1997—MS #744, Milwaukee, WI 53201.

E-mail address: rschum@mcw.edu

0031-3955/07/$ - see front matter © 2007 Elsevier Inc. All rights reserved.
doi:10.1016/j.pcl.2007.02.010

Atypical development of language can be classified as disordered or delayed. Delayed language will progress in a typical sequence, but at a slower rate than is normal. In contrast, disordered language has a different quality as it emerges. Certain language structures might appear out of order from the typical pattern of development. For example, a child can speak a well-formed sentence, but cannot answer "wh-" questions. Or, for another example, the child can comprehend an "if ..., then ..." conditional from a parent, but cannot properly use pronouns. The distinction between delayed and disordered language is often helpful in differential diagnosis of developmental disorders.

Delayed and disordered language can occur as a primary condition, such as a language disorder or a specific language impairment (SLI). Atypical language development is also a secondary characteristic of other physical and developmental problems that are often first manifested by language problems. These include hearing loss, mental retardation, autistic spectrum disorders, and learning disabilities. Speech problems can signal a specific physical disorder, such as speech apraxia (ie, a coordination disorder of speech articulators) or dysarthria (ie, impaired muscular function in speech production), or other neuromuscular disorders (eg, cerebral palsy) that affect speech production. Some children will show a phonological disorder that affects their ability to process speech sounds. Speech production problems can occur independently of language. Some children who have apraxia, phonological disorders, or cerebral palsy have typical language development. On the other hand, these speech disorders can co-occur with language difficulties. A combined speech and language delay occurs in 5% to 8% of preschool-aged children [2]. The majority of preschool-aged children who have language problems continue to show some form of language problem or learning difficulty throughout their childhood years, whether or not they receive intervention [3–6].

Hearing loss that is severe enough to affect language development and learning occurs in 1 to 6 per 1000 children [7]. Hearing loss will typically cause a delay in language development, rather than a disorder, during the early years of a child. Children who have hearing loss might have a reduced rate of vocabulary development, and continue to show delays in development of syntax and expanded phrases. Furthermore, they sometimes show distortions of speech sounds and prosody patterns. For these reasons, a child presenting with atypical articulation or rhythm of speech may have hearing loss, in addition to, or as a cause of, a speech disorder.

Children who have mental retardation will show a delay in development of language. Children who have mild cognitive impairment will use speech as preschoolers, but manifest delays in vocabulary development and the use of phrases. Children who have more severe impairment sometimes do not use words during their preschool years [8,9].

Children who have autistic spectrum disorders usually show a pattern of language disorder as a key component of their impairment. They may have phonological, syntactic, semantic, or pragmatic impairments. The diagnosis of autism requires three criteria: impaired communication, impaired social interaction, and repetitive behaviors/circumscribed interests. Some young autistic children will not express any words and have limited receptive language. Others might show a disordered pattern of language. For example, they might use echolalia (ie, repeating verbatim what others have said), but cannot generate their own novel phrases. Children who have autism, even if they do well in the systematic domains of language (phonology, syntax, semantics), nevertheless commonly show significant pragmatic difficulties in their inability to initiate or sustain a conversation. It is noteworthy that approximately three fourths of autistic children also have mental retardation [10]. Therefore, autistic children who have co-occurring mental retardation might be delayed in using any expressive language, whereas autistic children who have milder cognitive impairment might speak, but show a disordered pattern of language.

Language disorders can be a primary problem that is a separate and unique condition. It is variously referred to as an expressive or mixed receptive-expressive language disorder [11], or an SLI [12]. Language disorders are often implicated in subsequent learning disabilities, such as dyslexia. Prevalence studies indicate that one third to one half of school-aged children who have SLI also have reading disorders [13]. Furthermore, approximately one half of children who have psychiatric disorders also have language impairments [14,15]. A pediatrician should think about the possibility of a language delay/disorder whenever a child presents with significant behavioral problems.

Warning signs

A toddler or preschool child who has a language disorder might often be first identified in a pediatrician's office during a well-child check. Some parents might worry that their child has a hearing loss or a speech delay, and voice their concerns to the pediatrician. These are often parents who have older children, or who have had other experiences around young children, and therefore have a tacit sense of typical language development in children. They might comment that the child seems to have "selective hearing," in that sometimes the child responds to what is said and other times does not. Other parents, who do not have as much experience with young children, might not voice any concerns about communication delay. In this second situation, the pediatrician might be the first to note an atypical pattern of communication during a well-child examination.

The following seven clinical case descriptions illustrate how children who have atypical language development might present in the pediatrician's office.

Case 1: the child who has delayed onset of words

One situation is that of a child who does not use any words, or even word approximations, at 15 months of age. Sometimes the parents will realize that this represents a delay in language development. They might contrast this child's delay in using words with the language development of older siblings or cousins. They may understand the general rule of thumb to expect first words around the first birthday. Sometimes the parents do not immediately recognize the delay, but reveal it in discussion with the pediatrician who is reviewing the child's development. In retrospect, the parents report that the child did not coo or babble much during infancy. The parents might have described this child as a quiet baby who was not fussy or demanding.

Case 2: the shy toddler

A second scenario is of a toddler (18–24 months of age) who seems shy in the pediatrician's office. The child might not talk to the pediatrician, and might not respond to requests such as, "Show me your nose." It is important that the pediatrician not dismiss this as shyness during a medical examination. Rather, the pediatrician should inquire if this behavior is typical for what the child is like at home. If this lack of communication is typical for the child's behavior at home, then the child's behavior does not represent shyness, but more likely represents a significant communication delay. In contrast, the parents may report that the child's use of speech and language at home is consistent with typical development, such as using 100 to 200 words and combining them in short phrases. In this variation, the pediatrician should further interview the parents to determine if the reticence to talk seems specific to the medical appointment, or if the child shows a more generalized reticence to speak when outside the household, including with more familiar persons such as extended family members. If the reticence is specific to the medical visit, the pediatrician can monitor the child's progress over the next several visits. If the reticence seems generalized, the pediatrician might want to consider the possibility of selective mutism, and refer the child to a mental health practitioner for an evaluation [16].

Case 3: the child who gestures but does not speak

This is a situation of a child who uses gestures but not words. The child might use extensive gestures such as nodding/shaking the head, pointing, shrugging, and showing objects. Some children even include sound effects to signify objects, but not use words. The gesturing suggests that the child is motivated to communicate, but lacks expressive ability. This pattern can be suggestive of a motor speech disorder, such as apraxia, or of a hearing loss.

Case 4: the child who does not seem to understand words

Another scenario is of a child who does not seem to hear or listen. The child does not turn to look when a person calls the child's name and does not inhibit when admonished, "No!" Parents may speculate that the child is willfully ignoring them, or that the child has an "attention problem"; however, over time they notice that the child does not seem to recognize other words, even when the child is attentive to the parents. For example, the child does not seem to recognize or look at objects or people named by the parents. Obviously, a first hypothesis for this is hearing loss; however, some children will show this pattern even after a recent hearing examination reveals normal hearing acuity. This situation is suggestive of a receptive language problem or mental retardation.

Case 5: the child who has language regression

Some children will present with a history of language regression. Parents will report to the pediatrician that the child was saying words between 12 and 18 months, and then stopped saying words. Language regression is sometimes implicated in autism. About one fourth of autistic children show developmental regression between 15 and 21 months [17]. This includes loss of words (usually at the stage of the first 10 words), and regression of other social interests. One must be careful in interpreting this type of regression, however; a careful interview of the parents might indicate that the child had a history of atypical development, including in social interaction, before the regression, and that the few words that were used and then lost might not have be used meaningfully. Furthermore, there are no systematic studies that compare prevalence of regression among children who have autism, specific language impairment, and mental retardation. This early type of language regression might suggest some type of atypical development, but it has not been proven to be a unique and specific indicator of autism [18]. In contrast, a more severe pattern of regression occurs with a smaller group of autistic children (approximately 8%) after the second birthday, and includes the loss of phrases of two or more words. This more profound regression is associated with autism and disintegrative disorders such as Rett syndrome and childhood disintegrative disorder [17].

Case 6: the child who uses echolalia

Sometimes a pediatrician will meet a preschooler who uses echolalia, which is repeating verbatim what someone else has said. With immediate echolalia, the child repeats back what has just been said. With delayed echolalia, the child repeats a phrase, sentence, or even a passage that was previously heard, such as a line from a favorite movie. Echolalia is not unique to autism, but frequently represents disordered language. Younger children who have typically developing language commonly use short holistic phrases (eg, uttering a formulaic phrase without any type of grammatical analysis). For example, when children acquire a 100-word vocabulary, this includes about 20 phrases [19]. Children who have disordered language often show a pattern of syntactic impairment, however. They have difficulty analyzing the grammar of messages that come to them, and they have difficultly building grammatically sound expressive utterances. In lieu of their own unique phrases, they might substitute memorized, holistic phrases. This over-dependence on holistic phrases is a marker of atypical, disordered language. Children who have various language-based disorders demonstrate this, including children who have specific language impairment or autism.

Case 7: the child who has suspected hearing loss

A child may present with suspected hearing loss. The American Academy of Pediatrics recommends that if a parent is concerned that a child cannot hear, the pediatrician should assume that this concern is true until the child can be fully evaluated [7]. With the advent of neonatal hearing screening, many congenital hearing problems are identified at birth. In the United States, 45 states and the District of Columbia have legally mandated or voluntary compliance programs to screen newborn hearing [20]. Not all childhood hearing loss can be identified at newborn screening, however, because of the less than 100% accuracy of screening tests, because of progressive hearing loss, and because of acquired hearing loss caused by known or unknown etiology [7,21]. Post-lingual hearing loss (ie, hearing loss after spoken language is established) is sometimes difficult to pick up at first, because it often has a gradual effect on language. Signs of progressive post-lingual hearing loss include a parent report that the child does not seem to be listening, a gradual decline in the precision of speech articulation, a lack of progress in vocabulary acquisition, and a pattern of the child speaking better than listening.

Screening measures for language development

The US Preventive Services Task Force evaluated the use of brief, formal screening instruments for speech and language delays in young children that can be used in a primary care setting [1,2]. The Task Force focused on measures which require 10 minutes or less to complete—a necessary criterion in busy clinical settings. The results indicated that there was no sufficient evidence that screening instruments are any more reliable or effective than using physician observations or parental concerns to identify children who need further evaluation. The Task Force noted that there is no single "gold standard" for screening, because measures and terminology are used inconsistently. The Task Force recommended further research in this area, but did not recommend the use of screening instruments. It noted that in clinical evaluations, the most salient risk factors for speech and language problems include family history of speech/language delay, male gender, and perinatal factors. Family history should cover three generations to include siblings, parents, and grandparents. Speech/language delays in relatives might present in different variations, including late talkers, learning disabilities, dyslexia, special education services, history of speech therapy, or stuttering. Perinatal factors include preterm, low birth weight, birth difficulties, toxemia, and poor sucking [2].

Many of the formal screening measures are compilations of items from more extensive developmental inventories. It appears that the creators of the instruments tried to identify the most salient items for the screening measures. The Task Force determined that the use of the formal measures was not time or cost efficient, and deferred to pediatrician and parent concerns as indicators of potential problems. This leaves the question of what are reasonable indicators for a pediatrician's clinical evaluation of a child. Table 1 offers guidelines for raising concerns and referring a child to a specialist for further evaluation. Items for this chart were taken from four sources of normal development of language skills: Denver Developmental Screening Test II [22], the Rossetti Infant-Toddler Language Scale [23], and schedules of language development from the American Speech-Language-Hearing Association [24] and the Child Development Institute [25]. Table 1 identifies items at age levels that exceed norms by 25% to 50%, as well as adding noteworthy clinical features of echolalia and regression.

Referrals

Children's speech and language can be evaluated at any age when there is a suspicion of delay or disorder. The most common referral is to a speech-language pathologist for an evaluation. Some speech-language services, such as at a hospital or clinic, might have audiological services associated with them. In such settings, a hearing examination is part of the assessment protocol. If the speech-language service does not have audiology services available, or if the pediatrician suspects that hearing loss is the primary problem, then the pediatrician should make a direct referral to an audiologist or an otologist for a hearing evaluation.

The US federal IDEA law (Individuals with Disabilities Education Act) requires that special education services be provided to children who have learning difficulties, including those who have speech, language, and hearing problems. Each state has its own procedures for implementing that law, but has services available for children from birth to 21 years of age. The early intervention services in a particular state can provide speech-language evaluations of toddlers and preschoolers upon parent request. This is an appropriate resource for a pediatrician who suspects atypical language development. In addition, speech-language pathologists are available at

Table 1
Speech-language screening for pediatricians

Should absolutely refer for a speech-language evaluation if:		
At age	Receptive	Expressive
15 months	Does not look/point at 5–10 objects/ people named by parent	Not using three words
18 months	Does not follow simple directions ("Get your shoes.")	Not using Mama, Dada, or other names
24 months	Does not point to pictures or body parts when they are named	Not using 25 words
30 months	Does not verbally respond or nod/shake head to questions	Not using unique two-word phrases, including noun-verb combinations
36 months	Does not understand prepositions or action words; does not follow two-step directions	Vocabulary <200 words; does not ask for things by name; echolalia to questions; regression of language after acquiring two-word phrases

hospitals, clinics, and in private practice. They have standard methods for assessing language difficulties, and can make recommendations regarding treatment and intervention. This early intervention is available through the state education system. In addition, some children can obtain private therapy services.

Early intervention for speech and language problems is often effective in improving communication skills, when compared with no treatment [2]. A meta-analysis of treatment with young children who have speech and language difficulties, and no co-occurring conditions, shows promising results [26]. Children who have expressive phonological or language difficulties show significant improvement with treatment. There is mixed evidence for the efficacy of treatment for children who have expressive syntax problems, although it appears that intervention for this type of problem is more effective if the child does not also have receptive language difficulties. Current evidence is inconclusive for the efficacy of treatment with children who have receptive phonology or language problems. Interventions of longer duration (>8 weeks) appear to be more effective than interventions of shorter duration.

Parent counseling

A pediatrician who identifies atypical language development in a child will need to discuss this concern, and an appropriate referral, with the child's parents. In this context, the pediatrician counsels the parents about the suspected problem and how it should be managed. The goals of such counseling are to provide hope and information. Hope focuses on reassuring the parents that there are things they can do to improve their child's situation. The pediatrician can reassure the parents that there are professionals and services available to their child, so the parents do not have to face this alone. The goal of information is to help the parents have a clear understanding of their child's problem, while minimizing any misunderstanding or misinterpretation of the situation.

In meeting the information goal, the pediatrician should be careful not to prematurely diagnose the child's problem before the child has had a thorough evaluation by a specialist. For example, because autism is such a publicly recognized disorder, it is a common mistake for parents, and some professionals, to assume that an early language disorder automatically signals autism. The lay public has been sensitized to autistic symptoms, which include communication problems; however, the public is less well-versed on other developmental disorders that also have language impairment as a symptom, such as mental retardation and specific language impairment. If possible, the pediatrician should focus the discussion on the behaviors of the child, rather than the diagnosis of the child. Talk with the parents about verbs—what the child does—rather than nouns—what the child is. The pediatrician can express concern about the child's behaviors (ie, problems with language), and can talk to the parents about the need for further evaluation by specialists. As much as possible, the pediatrician should defer differential diagnosis to the specialists.

If the parents bring up concerns about a specific diagnosis, such as autism, then the pediatrician can expand their range of information. For example, the pediatrician might confirm that the language disorder could possibly reflect autism, but that there are other disorders that are also associated with disordered language. The point is to help the parents stay open to various possibilities and not become prematurely set in understanding the child's difficulty in one particular way. The pediatrician can explain other possible diagnoses that might be in play. Although it can be unsettling for parents to hear of the possibility of mental retardation, this is unlikely to be any less upsetting than a diagnosis of autism. If the parents can consider the possibility of autism, then they can hear alternatives that include other significant impairments.

Following the child's development over time is an important diagnostic tool for counseling parents. The child's changes and response to intervention over time can clarify the scope and persistence of the child's problems. As the child's communication skills improve, one can determine if other behavioral or developmental problems persist, or if these co-occurring problems improve along with the communication. For example, a child's social behavior is often linked with the level of communication facility [27]. A young child's social isolation may appear to be a primary disorder, such as attributable to autism; however, as the child's communication improves, the child might have more skills to expand on social opportunities with adults and children. If social behavior and interests improve with communication progress, this argues against a primary social deficit seen in autistic disorders. Furthermore, recognition of this social behavior-communication link can help parents understand why their child behaves in a certain way, and can help them learn more effective techniques in managing behavior problems (eg, use management techniques adjusted to communication level rather than chronological age).

The child's periodic visits with the pediatrician afford an opportunity for the pediatrician to review the child's rate of progress with the parents. During these reviews, it is helpful to note the child's intra-individual changes since the previous visit, and not merely focus on the child's current status compared with age-based norms. This focuses on the positive growth of the child, rather than accentuating the child's continuing differences with typical development.

With the other counseling goal of hope, the pediatrician can also focus on verbs, what parents can do to help their child, rather than nouns, what their child is. Many parents are anxious and concerned for their child. The pediatrician can reduce anxiety by giving parents activities to bind their anxiety into constructive action. For example, a pediatrician can recommend a parent-friendly book, *The New Language of Toys* [28]. This book gives parents practical ideas on how to use toys and books in a developmentally appropriate manner to stimulate communication with their children. It provides many specific suggestions, and offers developmental guidelines to help parents understand where their child's developmental skills fall in a sequence. Another helpful book for parents is *Childhood Speech, Language, and Listening Problems* [29], which explains different communication problems and advises parents on resources that are available for helping their child. By recommending books such as these, the pediatrician provides hope to parents by giving them positive activities, so they can do something to improve their child's problem.

Hope is also offered by reassuring parents that they are not alone in their quest to determine what is wrong with their child and how to improve that situation. The pediatrician can explain that with a referral, the parents will meet knowledgeable specialists who will help the parents further investigate the language problem. The pediatrician can explain to the parents that there are a variety of services and programs available for children who have communication problems, and that children often improve in their communication abilities. Wise pediatricians do not offer false hope—that everything will be okay. Rather, they offer the realistic hope that there are professionals who can work with the children and parents, after an appropriate diagnosis is made, and that many times the children show positive response to such programs.

Summary

In summary, atypical language development is an important symptom of a variety of developmental difficulties. At the present time, parent and pediatrician impressions of atypical communication are as good an indicator of problems as any type of formal screening measure. A pediatrician should be aware of the range of problems that can be represented by a language disorder, and subsequent articles discuss these implications in more detail. The pediatrician is usually the lead person in spotting atypical development. Whenever a communication disorder is suspected, children are old enough for an evaluation by specialists. Early intervention with speech and language therapy is often effective in helping to improve a child's communication disorder. Pediatricians can effectively counsel parents by using the guiding principles of providing hope and information.

References

[1] US Preventive Services Task Force. Screening for speech and language delay in preschool children: recommendation statement. Pediatrics 2006;117:497–501.

[2] Nelson HD, Nygren P, Walker M, et al. Screening for speech and language delay in preschool children: systematic evidence review for the US Preventive Services Task Force. Pediatrics 2006;117:e298–319.

[3] Aram D, Nation J. Preschool language disorders and subsequent language and academic difficulties. J Commun Disord 1980;13:159–70.

[4] Aram D, Ekelman B, Nation J. Preschoolers with language disorders: 10 years later. J Speech Hear Res 1984;27:232–44.

[5] Bishop D, Edmundson A. Language impaired 4-year-olds: distinguishing transient from persistent impairment. J Speech Hear Disord 1987;52:156–73.

[6] Beitchman J, Brownlie E, Inglis A, et al. Seven-year follow-up of speech/language-impaired and control children: speech/language stability and outcome. J Am Acad Child Adolesc Psychiatry 1994;33(9):1322–30.

[7] Cunningham M, Cox EO; Committee on Practice and Ambulatory Medicine, and the Section of Otolaryngology and Bronchoesophagology. Hearing assessment in infants and children: recommendations beyond neonatal screening. Pediatrics 2003;111(2):436–40.

[8] McCathren RB, Yoder PJ, Warren SF. The relationship between prelinguistic vocalization and later expressive vocabulary in young children with developmental delay. J Speech Hear Res 1999;42:915–24.

[9] Romski M, Sevcik RA, Fonseca AH. Augmentative and alternative communication for persons with mental retardation. In: Abbeduto L, editor. Language and communication in mental retardation. International review of research in mental retardation, vol . 27. San Diego (CA): Academic Press; 2003. p. 255–80.

[10] Siegel B. Helping children with autism learn. New York: Oxford; 2003.

[11] American Psychiatric Association. Diagnostic and statistical manual of mental disorders. 4th edition. Washington, DC: American Psychiatric Association; 1994.

[12] Leonard LB. Children with specific language impairment. Cambridge (MA): MIT Press; 1998.

[13] Catts HW, Adlof SM, Hogan TP, et al. Are specific language impairment and dyslexia distinct disorders? J Speech Hear Res 2005;48:1378–96.

[14] Cohen NJ, Davine M, Horodezky N, et al. Unsuspected language impairment in psychiatrically disturbed children: prevalence and language and behavioral characteristics. J Am Acad Child Adolesc Psychiatry 1993;32:595–603.

[15] Cohen NJ, Horodezky NB. Language impairments and psychopathology. J Am Acad Child Adolesc Psychiatry 1998;37:461–2.

[16] Schum R. Clinical perspectives on the treatment of selective mutism. The Journal of Speech-Language Pathology and Applied Behavior Anaylsis 2006;1(2):149–63.

[17] Baird G, Cass H, Slonims V. Diagnosis of autism. BMJ 2003;327:488–93.

[18] Rutter M. Autism: its recognition, early diagnosis, and service implications. J Dev Behav Pediatr 2006;27(2 Suppl):S54–8.

[19] Locke JL. A theory of neurolinguistic development. Brain Lang 1997;58:265–326.

[20] American Speech-Hearing-Language Association. ASHA Leader September 3: 23; 2006.

[21] Lutman ME, Davis AC, Fortnum HM, et al. Field sensitivity of targeted neonatal hearing screening by transient-evoked otoacoustic emissions. Ear Hear 1997;18(4):265–76.

[22] Frankenburg WK, Dodds J, Archer P, et al. The Denver II: a major revision and restandard-ization of the Denver developmental screening test. Pediatrics 1992;89(1):91–7.

[23] Rossetti L. The Rossetti Infant-Toddler Language Scale. East Moline (IL): LinguiSystems; 1990.

[24] American Speech-Language-Hearing Association. How does your child hear and talk? 2006. Available at: http://asha.org/public/speech/development/child_hear_talk.htm. Accessed September 19, 2006.

[25] Child Development Institute. Language development in children. 2005. Available at: http://www.childdevelopmentinfo.com/development/language_development.shtml. Accessed May 30, 2006.

[26] Law J, Garrett Z, Nye C. The efficacy of treatment for children with developmental speech and language delay/disorder: a meta-analysis. J Speech Hear Res 2004;47:924–43.

[27] Schum R. Communication and social growth: a developmental model of social behavior in deaf children. Ear Hear 1991;12(5):320–7.

[28] Schwartz S. The new language of toys: teaching communication skills to children with special needs. Bethesda (MD): Woodbine House; 1996.

[29] Hamaguchi PM. Childhood speech, language, and listening problems. New York: Wiley; 1995.

ELSEVIER
SAUNDERS

PEDIATRIC CLINICS
OF NORTH AMERICA

Pediatr Clin N Am 54 (2007) 437–467

Language Disorders in Children: Classification and Clinical Syndromes

Mark D. Simms, MD, MPH[a,b],*

[a]Section of Developmental Pediatrics, Department of Pediatrics, Medical
College of Wisconsin, 8701 Watertown Plank Road, Milwaukee, WI 53226, USA
[b]Child Development Center, Children's Hospital of Wisconsin, PO Box 1997,
Mail Station 744, Milwaukee, WI 53226–1997, USA

Language development is a central feature of cognitive and social development in humans. A principal purpose of language is to mediate interactions between individuals. Language also helps us to understand the world and our experiences in it. Words provide a means to learn new concepts and organize thoughts. According to Pinker [1], development of language is instinctual:

Language is not a cultural artifact that we learn the way we learn to tell time or how the federal government works. Instead, it is a distinct piece of the biological makeup of our brains. Language is a complex, specialized skill, which develops in the child spontaneously, without conscious effort or formal instruction, is deployed without awareness of its underlying logic, is qualitatively the same in every individual, and is distinct from more general abilities to process information and behavior intelligently.

When language fails to develop naturally, however, the consequences are widespread and potentially severe.

Communication disorders are among the most common developmental problems encountered in general pediatrics. The prevalence of language delay in children varies with age. At 24 months of age, up to 17% of children are thought to have delayed onset of talking [2]. The causes of such delayed development are varied. Poor speech or language development are often associated with chronic physical health problems (eg, cerebral palsy, epilepsy, cleft lip and palate); mental retardation; birth defect syndromes; social and environmental disadvantage; or autism spectrum disorders. Of these comorbid conditions, mental retardation is the most common. In one study of

* Child Development Center, Children's Hospital of Wisconsin, PO Box 1997, Mail Station 744, Milwaukee, WI 53226–1997.
  E-mail address: msimms@mcw.edu

0031-3955/07/$ - see front matter © 2007 Elsevier Inc. All rights reserved.
doi:10.1016/j.pcl.2007.02.014
pediatric.theclinics.com

language-delayed 3 year olds (whose language age was less than two thirds of their chronologic age), 37% were also delayed in nonverbal mental abilities [3]. By kindergarten entry, approximately 7.4% of children are thought to have a language development disorder not related to mental retardation [4].

Language typically develops in a very predictable fashion, and assessment of language development should be a central part of every well-child visit. Pediatricians are in an excellent position to identify children's speech and language problems early and to make appropriate referrals for further evaluation and treatment services.

Brief overview of normal language development

Acquisition of communication and language abilities proceeds from preverbal to verbal skills; comprehension of language information precedes use of spoken words. By the end of the second trimester, the fetus can perceive its mother's voice. Soon after birth, infants begin to discriminate speech sounds. Nonverbal skills that set the stage for communication also emerge soon after birth. Attention to an adult's tone of voice, facial expression, and body movements is present by 3 months of age. Imitation and reciprocal vocal exchanges emerge by 6 months. Social gesture games ("peek-a-boo," "so-big," and "bye-bye") are typically well established by 9 to 10 months of age. Many toddlers demonstrate understanding of words by pointing selectively on request or through other behavioral means before they are able to say words. Expressively, word labels (true words) are acquired though a process of imitation and are used in a variety of communicative ways. Once the infant is able to use between 50 and 75 true words, two-word phrases appear. The ability to combine words reflects an understanding of grammar (syntax). Although primitive at first, this quickly becomes rather complex. By age 3 years, many children are able to use three-word sentences with correct word order, personal pronouns, and simple past tense forms of regular verbs. At least half of what a 3 year old says (speech articulation) should be intelligible to a stranger. By 5 years, most children are able to answer open-ended questions, such as when, why, and how. Conversational skills allow them to hold a short conversation with connected sentences, maintain a topic, and use language to acquire information and regulate their behavior. Speech is largely intelligible to strangers. As development of communication skills proceeds, children acquire increasingly sophisticated facility in understanding and using language to initiate and regulate social interactions. By age 7 to 8 years of age, children are able to understand and use complex sentence structures in everyday conversation, and they begin to grasp the subtleties of irony, sarcasm, and humor.

Elements of language

A variety of terms describe elements of language when evaluating a child's communication abilities. At the most basic level, individual sounds that are used to form spoken words are called "phonemes." Each language, and each dialect within a given language, uses different sets of phonemes. "Morphology" refers to the units of language that are appended to words to express an attribute. For example, English morphemes include grammatical inflections to indicate possessives, case, or verb tense. Rules of grammar, or syntax, determine the way words are combined to form meaningful sentences. "Semantics" refers to the specific meaning of words, phrases, and sentences. The rhythm, intonation, and modulation of pitch in words, groups of words, or sentences that communicate the speaker's intentions constitute "vocal prosody." Finally, "pragmatics" refers to the appropriate use of verbal and nonverbal components of communication. Key aspects of verbal pragmatics include initiating, joining, and ending conversations, and providing sufficient contextual references for one's communicative partner. Nonverbal pragmatics includes eye contact, facial expression, body posture, and gestures. Individual components of language generally work together to create effective communication. Children with good pragmatic abilities are often able to compensate for weak grammar or word knowledge.

Definition and classification of communication disorders

There have been many attempts to describe and classify disorders of language development [5]. None, however, has gained universal clinical application. The American Psychiatric Association's *Diagnostic and Statistical Manual* (DSM-IV) provides a very basic classification system for disorders of language and communication.

DSM-IV [6] recognizes three types of communication disorders: (1) expressive, (2) mixed receptive-expressive, and (3) phonologic and stuttering disorder (Box 1). Stuttering disorder is not included for the purposes of this discussion. These definitions include several key diagnostic considerations that are important to clinicians. First, communication disorders are characterized by a substantial discrepancy between language and nonverbal intellectual development, although no specific cutoff criteria are provided. In research settings, strict discrepancy criteria are used to distinguish individuals whose language impairments stem from specific problems with language ability from those whose problems are rooted in a general disorder of cognitive function. For example, specific language impairment (SLI) is usually defined by a combination of normal intelligence (performance intelligence quotient [IQ] ≥ 85) and language impairment (a composite language measure that falls more than 1.25 SD below the mean) [7]. This corresponds to the lower tenth percentile, a level at which speech-language clinicians typically identify a child as having a language impairment [8]. Typically, children with global developmental delays do not show significant discrepancies between language abilities and development in other domains, such as nonverbal intelligence, self-help, and social and motor skills. In practical terms, however, and according to DSM-IV criteria, it should be possible to

Box 1. DSM-IV classification of communication disorders

315.31 Expressive language disorder

A. The scores obtained from standardized individually administered measure of expressive language development are substantially below those obtained from standardized measures of both nonverbal intellectual capacity and receptive language development. The disturbance may be manifest clinically by symptoms that include having a markedly limited vocabulary, making errors in tense, or having difficulty recalling words or producing sentences with developmentally appropriate length or complexity.

B. The difficulties with expressive language interfere with academic or occupational achievement or with social communication.

C. Criteria are not met for mixed receptive-expressive language disorder or a pervasive developmental disorder.

D. If mental retardation, a speech-motor or sensory deficit, or environmental deprivation is present, the language difficulties are in excess of those usually associated with these problems.

315.31 Mixed receptive-expressive language disorder

A. The scores obtained from a battery of standardized individually administered measures of both receptive and expressive language development are substantially below those obtained from standardized measures of nonverbal intellectual capacity. Symptoms include those for expressive language disorder and difficulty understanding words; sentences; or specific types of words, such as spatial terms.

B. The difficulties with receptive and expressive language significantly interfere with academic or occupational achievement or with social communication.

C. Criteria are not met for a pervasive developmental disorder.

D. If mental retardation, a speech-motor or sensory deficit, or environmental deprivation is present, the language difficulties are in excess of those usually associated with these problems.

315.39 Phonologic disorder

A. Failure to use developmentally expected speech sounds that are appropriate for age and dialect (eg, errors in sound production, use, representation, or organization, such as, but not limited to, substitutions of one sound for another [use of/t/for target/k/sound] or omissions of sounds, such as final consonants).

B. The difficulties in speech sound production interfere with academic or occupational achievement or with social communication.

C. If mental retardation, a speech-motor or sensory deficit, or environmental deprivation is present, the speech difficulties are in excess of those usually associated with these problems.

identify disordered language development even in individuals with low general intelligence [9].

A second consideration in the definition of communication disorder involves exclusionary criteria. In research settings, individuals with low IQ, hearing loss, prematurity, neurologic disease, genetic disorders, environmental deprivation, emotional disturbances, and pervasive developmental disorder (eg, autism) are excluded from the study group. In clinical practice, however, children with these excluded comorbid disorders often show language deficits similar to those who meet the stricter research definition of SLI. Alternatively, many of the children with the excluded conditions do not exhibit language impairment. DSM-IV accepts the diagnosis of communication disorder in a wide range of comorbid conditions as long as language difficulties are "in excess of those usually associated with these problems."

Third, from a clinical perspective, DSM-IV definitions include the provision that language difficulties must interfere with academic or occupational achievement or with social communication. The presence of a communication disorder is not simply a statistical definition based on standardized test scores. As noted later, some higher-level aspects of communication involving social use of language (pragmatics) have not yet been adequately quantified through standardized testing.

Finally, language abilities clearly change with age, and in children with language impairments patterns of language difficulty can vary quite markedly as they grow older. Children with SLI typically are behind their peers in both quantitative and qualitative measures of language ability.

In clinical practice, identification of children with SLI usually incorporates elements of both a discrepancy between verbal and nonverbal cognitive abilities, and evaluation of the pattern of language development and current usage. Further, there is often considerable variation within an individual child's profile of language abilities, and evidence of a nontypical sequence of acquisition of language skills, as described later. To a large extent, diagnosis of communication disorders relies on a combination of objective test data and clinical acumen.

Clinical characteristics

Within the broad context of the DSM-IV classification scheme, clinicians are likely to encounter children with a wide range of language and communication difficulties.

Isolated expressive language disorder

By definition, children with isolated expressive language disorder have normal nonverbal cognitive ability and age-appropriate understanding of spoken language but are limited in their ability to talk. Often, they seem to have a small vocabulary and they have difficulty learning new words. Word retrieval deficits may also be present and manifest with nonverbal "place holders" (eg, frequent use of "uhmm"), or nondescript verbal substitutions (eg, referring to specific objects as "that thing"). Sentences may be short; grammatical structures simplified; and certain classes of words may be omitted, such as articles ("a," "the," and so forth). Lacking command of normal syntactic forms, the child may link together a string of short phrases rather than make a series of complete sentences. It is important to distinguish whether the child's limited spoken language is the result of a speech production difficulty or a reflection of an underlying expressive language deficit (or both). In very young children, whose speech is limited, assessment of articulation may be difficult. If speech sound production is adequate, however, the child may have an isolated expressive language disorder.

Mixed receptive-expressive language disorder (specific language impairment)

According to Bishop [10], "There are children who are physically and emotionally intact, who have been raised in homes with articulate, loving, communicative parents, and whose development is following a normal course in all other areas, but for whom language learning poses major problems." Many diagnostic and descriptive terms have been applied to this condition, including "developmental aphasia," "developmental dysphasia," "delayed language," "specific developmental language disorder," and SLI.

In general, young children with SLI resemble other children who are "late talkers." They typically utter their first words later, and combine words later, than their peers. Once they begin speaking, their language is characterized by a smaller vocabulary of words, and they tend to use fewer complex expressions that contain more grammatical errors than one would expect to see in children of that age. Children with language impairment may have difficulty with time concepts, such as yesterday, tomorrow, or after. They may use language that is vague, nonspecific, and lacks detail, substituting "that thing" or "stuff" in place of specific objects.

An inability to process phonologic aspects of language efficiently is strongly correlated with limited word knowledge. As a result, these children cannot map meaning to recurrent strings of sounds from incoming speech information. For example, when asked to repeat nonsense words (a task that simply requires processing of speech sounds, not word meaning) children with SLI experience particular difficulty with nonwords of greater than two syllables [11–13].

Another early language pattern seen in some children with SLI is echolalic memorization of phrases or dialog from movies or stories. Often, children use these echolalic phrases in appropriate contexts. This pattern likely reflects a specific weakness in the understanding and use of grammatical knowledge such that the children cannot spontaneously combine words to form sentences, even though they understand the overall meaning (gist) of the phrases. Reliance on repetition of large "chunks" of language reflects a holistic "top down" pattern of language development in children who do not know how to construct sentences appropriately from the "bottom up."

In SLI, some aspects of language cause greater problems than others, particularly grammar and phonology. Difficulty mastering the rules of grammar governing how words are arranged to make phrases and sentences typically leads to shorter and more simplified utterances. Compared with younger children, those with SLI show an uneven profile of language skills, with a pattern of errors that are uncommon in children with normal language development. As their language skills develop, there is a persistent and disproportionate impairment in the grammatical comprehension and expression of language [14].

Certain grammatical inflections (the markers applied to words to indicate a specific attribute) are very difficult for many children with SLI. For example, tense markings of verbs (ie, "he walked to school"), the possessive inflection/s/ (ie, "Bob's ball"), and the third-person singular inflection/s/ of regular verbs to indicate subject-verb agreement (ie, "she runs") are used incorrectly more often than the plural inflection/s/ (ie, "three cups"), which does not require understanding of syntactic rules.

Understanding and use of questions is typically mastered by age 4 years. Many children with SLI have great difficulty, however, with questions [15]. The grammatical complexity of a simple question form is apparent when considering the difference in structure and function between statements and questions. A simple question ("Is the ball under the chair?") differs from a statement ("The ball is under the chair") in at least three attributes: (1) word order of the verb-object is reversed, (2) the vocal inflection pattern ends in an up-swing, and (3) there is an implied request for an answer.

Grammatical knowledge is also needed for the assignment of reference to personal pronouns (him or her) and reflexives (himself) in certain types of sentences. For example, gender or number alone provides cues to determining proper reference for pronouns and reflexives. In the sentence, "The lady knew the boy was talking to her," gender determines that "her" refers to the lady. In other circumstances, however, correct interpretation of pronoun reference depends on understanding grammatical knowledge. At around 5 years of age, children correctly understand the references in the following sentences: "Baloo Bear says Mowgli is pointing to him. Baloo Bear says Mowgli is pointing to himself" [10].

In the first sentence, "him" has to refer to Baloo Bear. In the second sentence, "himself" has to refer to Mowgli. Children with SLI have great difficulty working out pronoun reference on the basis of grammatical information [10].

Higher-level language disorders

Pragmatic language disorder

Effective communication depends on mastery of skills that extend beyond basic understanding of words and rules of grammar and involves appropriate use of language in social settings. This aspect of communication is referred to as "pragmatics." By the time children enter school, they begin to understand and use idioms and humor. Conversational content also becomes more complex as children mature, as do communication demands placed on them. Between 7 and 9 years of age, children are able to interpret correctly tone of voice and facial expressions to judge a speaker's intentions. Teenagers are adept at the use of slang, metaphor, irony, and sarcasm. In one study, 11% of teachers' utterances in a typical fifth grade class contained at least one idiom. By seventh grade, this rose to approximately 20% [16]. The impact of weak pragmatic understanding becomes more apparent as children progress through school. Children are able to speak clearly and to use complex sentences; it is the inappropriateness or incoherence of their conversation that characterizes their pragmatic language disorder.

When first described, this condition was referred to as "semantic-pragmatic syndrome" in recognition of the contribution of poor semantics, or word meaning, to the breakdown of conversational abilities in affected children [5]. Children who have this disorder understand short phrases and individual words, but have difficulty comprehending the social context of conversations. In both Williams syndrome and in spina bifida complicated by hydrocephalus, children are often very fluent and use grammatically correct sentences, but their language is not effective in promoting social interaction. They may initiate long, rambling monologues or answer questions with seemingly irrelevant responses. Pinker [1] quotes an 18-year-old girl with Williams syndrome:

> And what an elephant is, it is one of the animals. And what the elephant does, it lives in the jungle. It can also live in the zoo. And what it has, it has long, gray ears, fan ears, ears that can blow in the wind. It has a long trunk that can pick up grass or pick up hay...If they're in a bad mood, it can be terrible...If the elephant gets mad, it could stomp; it could charge. Sometimes elephants can charge, like a bull can charge. They have big, long, tusks. They can damage a car...It could be dangerous. When they're in a pinch, when they're in a bad mood, it can be terrible. You don't want an elephant as a pet. You want a cat or a dog or a bird.

Symptoms of pragmatic difficulty may also include extreme literalness that is the product of failure to understand aspects of additional meaning that can be inferred from sentences without actually being encoded in them [17]. Lacking ability to understand the intentions of others, individuals with pragmatic deficits may not provide their conversational partners with a sufficient referential base to understand their statements.

Pragmatic language impairment often occurs in the context of SLI, but it has been recognized as a symptom of a number of other disorders, including autism and pervasive developmental disorder, Asperger's syndrome, nonverbal learning disability, and right-hemisphere brain damage [17]. Some also recognize pragmatic language disorder as a distinctive developmental language disorder and not solely a symptom of another condition, like autism.

Articulation disorders

Speech articulation typically develops gradually during preschool years. Between 5 and 10 months of age, infants show repetitive (canonical) babbling (eg, bababa, dididi). Babbling soon turns into a type of nonsense speech (jargon) that often has the tone and rhythm of human speech but does not contain real words. By their first birthday, most children start to say true words, and these are mixed into the jargon. By 3 years of age, both parents and strangers understand most children's speech requests.

Phonologic disorder

Speech problems that interfere with sound articulation are usually the result of a phonologic impairment. Approximately 7.5% of 3- to 11-year-old children have clinically significant speech sound distortions [18]. As infants, children with phonologic disorder babble at the normal age, and produce a wide range of vowel and consonant sounds. As they progress in speech development, they typically omit, substitute, or reduce consonants and clusters of sounds. Children with phonologic speech disorder are frequently unintelligible, although parents and siblings may be able to decipher the child's utterances and "translate" for strangers. Physical examination, with particular emphasis on craniofacial structures and oromotor function, typically shows no abnormalities.

There is considerable overlap between speech and language delays and disorders in children. Between 50% and 75% of young children with delayed speech development also have delayed expressive language development, and 10% to 40% have language comprehension delay.

Follow-up studies of speech-delayed children identified during preschool years have shown variable outcome with regard to speech, language, and academic outcomes. Although the speech patterns of many children normalize over time, up to 5% persist in having residual articulation delays into adulthood. Children who experience significant difficulty producing clear speech sounds may be bullied by peers and experience frustration or reluctance to speak [19].

Dysarthria

Neuromuscular disorders, such as cerebral palsy, myopathy, closed head injury, stroke, and so forth, may result in poor articulation. Cerebral palsy frequently results in weakness and impaired control of muscles for both speech and nonspeech functions, such as smiling, chewing, and swallowing. Poor coordination of respiration associated with cerebral palsy may interfere with speech production. Dysarthria may manifest as slurred words, distorted consonants and vowels, with slow, labored speech. Nasal resonance may vary because of poor velopharyngeal control. Early feeding difficulty may be caused by tongue thrusting, weak facial muscles, and either hypersensitive or decreased gag reflex.

Apraxia

The child with apraxia of speech, a severe neuromotor coordination disorder, may present in infancy with early feeding problems that reflect poor oral coordination. Babbling may be very limited, and these children are often described as having been "very quiet" as infants. The range and complexity of early sound production is often reduced compared with typically developing children. Their efforts to imitate sounds seem labored and ineffective. To communicate, these children may grunt or point. Symptoms of frustration are common, because the more they try to talk, the more difficulty they may encounter in pronouncing words clearly. Inconsistency of sound production is a hallmark of speech apraxia [20,21]. On occasion, the child may say a word clearly but cannot repeat it on command (Box 2). As speech intelligibility improves, children with apraxia may develop a form of dysfluency, such as prolonging vowels to "buy time" to organize the coordination of the next series of oral movements. They may also have difficulty with alternating hypernasality and hyponasality because of poor coordination of the velopharyngeal valving and oral movements necessary for connected speech. In some cases, poor motor coordination (apraxia) is limited to speech production; however, generalized motor incoordination may also be present and interfere with other activities of daily living, such as dressing and eating.

Apraxia of speech is more common in boys than girls (with gender ratios ranging from 2:1–9:1), and family history of affected children often reveals other close relatives with speech and language disorders [22]. The prevalence of apraxia of speech has been estimated at between 1 and 10 per 1000. It is believed to reflect a deficit of motor planning in the central nervous system because there is full range of motion of all articulatory structures, normal strength, and the ability to make sounds in isolation. No specific lesion or anatomic abnormality has yet been identified as a possible cause. Prognosis seems less favorable for this than for other articulatory disorders; however, many children seem to respond well to intensive speech therapy. It is not uncommon for children with apraxia of speech to continue to have speech difficulty into their adult years.

Maturational delay (late bloomer or late talker syndrome)

Children with delayed expressive language development, who have no evidence of motor speech disorder and whose receptive language abilities are

---

Box 2. Apraxia of speech

Early symptoms suggestive of apraxia
Poor coordination of sucking response
Very quiet baby
Little or no babbling, but vowel-like vocalizations may be heard
Limited differentiation of consonants and vowels in the babbling
    repertoire
Limited spontaneous imitation of syllables
Excessive drooling

Diagnostic criteria for apraxia[a]
1. Struggle, groping, and trial and error behavior on production
   of some or all phonemes
2. Inability volitionally to produce an isolated phoneme or
   sequence of phonemes that have been produced correctly on
   other occasions
3. Failure to achieve, on command, isolated and sequenced oral
   movements available at an automatic level
4. Speech development shows a deviant pattern
5. Unable to produce, on a diadochokinetic task, sounds
   produced correctly in isolation
6. Increased number of articulation errors with increased length
   of utterance
7. Inconsistent pattern of articulation errors

---

[a]*Adapted from* Shriberg LD, Aram DM, Kwiatkowski J. Developmental apraxia
of speech: I. Descriptive and theoretical perspectives. J Speech Lang Hear Res
1997;40:273–85.

---

normal, may have a maturational expressive language delay. This condition
is considered to be a "normal variant" of development, and is a diagnosis
made by exclusion. Maturational delay should only be considered after
other causes of expressive language delay have been ruled out. Caution
must be exercised in making this diagnosis, because several longitudinal
studies found less than half of late-talking preschool children have normal
language abilities by age 5 years [23,24].

Maturational delay is believed to be more common in boys than girls,
and to run in families. Once they start talking, children with this pattern
of language development continue to do well and there is little long-term
risk of speech, language, or learning impairment. Although the subject of recent popular culture works [25] and clinical descriptions [26], there has been
little scientific research on this condition [27].

Comorbid impairments

Motor

Many children identified as having language impairment also have associated motor function problems. For example, Webster and colleagues [28] noted that nearly half of children diagnosed with developmental language disorder at preschool age had delays in gross and fine motor domains on standardized tests at the time of school entry. Children with SLI have been shown to have difficulty with both timed and nontimed fine motor tasks [29]. For example, impaired performance on a simple thumb tapping task was more strongly correlated with speech than with language deficits, although children with either or both problems scored lower than nonaffected controls [30]. Hill [31] noted that children with language impairments had more difficulty imitating familiar (meaningful) single hand gestures than matched, non–language-impaired age-peers. Surprisingly, their performance in imitating meaningless gestures was largely error-free. The authors attributed this difference to the children's reliance on visual monitoring when copying novel gestures. When carefully examined, the motor skills of children with SLI were found to resemble those of chronologically younger children. The authors concluded that the motor impairments of SLI children represent a maturational delay in development rather than a specific "motor planning deficit," as might be seen in generalized motor apraxia. Physical examination of children with language-impairment often reveals a mild degree of low resting muscle tone and increased range of joint motion. Other clinical observations include delay in toilet training skills, likely because of general motor immaturity.

General cognitive deficits in specific language impairment

Although children with language impairments may have overall nonverbal abilities that fall within the average or higher ranges of cognitive ability, researchers have identified deficits in a number of specific cognitive domains. For example, Nelson and colleagues [32] found children with SLI to have difficulty encoding both verbal and nonverbal information. In particular, children with SLI were less efficient in processing visually presented discrimination-learning problems. Rapin [33] found children with language disorders tended to score greater than 1.5 SD below the mean on the Stanford Binet Bead Memory task, a test of visual memory. Overall performance on the composite motor domain of the Vineland Adaptive Behavior Scales, and on the Annett Pegboard, a test of handedness, was in the borderline range. Hick and colleagues [34] noted children with SLI to have impairments in both visuospatial short-term memory and verbal short-term memory tasks. The researchers could not exclude the effect of limited verbal rehearsal strategies on task performance in language-impaired children. Similarly, Bavin and colleagues [35] noted differences in the performance of children with SLI and age-matched control children in some spatiovisual memory tasks that were not specific to the language domain.

The common association of nonverbal cognitive and motor impairments in children with language disorders has prompted some authors to suggest that the term "specific" in "specific language disorder" is inappropriate and should be dropped [36]. In a study by Fernell and colleagues [37], 87% of preschoolers with moderate or severe language impairment subjected to a broad-based assessment procedure were found to have associated nonlanguage developmental problems.

Associated emotional and behavioral problems

As a rule of thumb, children's social and emotional development is correlated with language development. By age 3, children can understand simple explanations and use their emerging language skills to "negotiate" with adults. By age 4, social interactions with peers are largely mediated through verbal transactions. Parents and teachers frequently report that children with language delays relate better to younger children, who function at their language level, or to older children and adults, who can interpret their intentions, than to normally developing age peers.

Children with communication difficulties frequently exhibit social and behavioral problems [38–41]. In a study of more than 300 children referred to an urban speech and language clinic, Cantwell and Baker [42] found that nearly half had emotional and behavioral disorders. The most common diagnoses in their sample were attention deficit disorder (19%); anxiety disorders (10%); and externalizing disorders (eg, oppositional defiant and conduct disorders [7%]). The prevalence of psychiatric disorder varied by type of speech or language problem. The highest rate (81%) was seen in children with language comprehension disorder, and the lowest rate (30%) was in those with isolated speech disorder. Beitchman and colleagues [43] noted similar findings in a representative community sample of 5-year-old children. Those with low overall language abilities (both expressive and receptive impairments) seemed to be the most disturbed, showing symptoms consistent with attention-deficit/hyperactivity disorder. In contrast, children whose primary problem involved poor articulation were the least disturbed on measures of behavioral and social competence.

A high rate of both diagnosed and undiagnosed language disorders has been identified in children seen in psychiatric clinics. Cohen and colleagues [44] found symptoms of SLI in 53% of a group of 399 children referred to three mental health clinics in Toronto. Almost half of these children had previously unsuspected language disorders. As noted by Cohen and Horodezky [45] and by Berk [46], children who experience difficulty processing language may be at a disadvantage because they possess poor verbal mediation skills with which to regulate their behavior, rehearse rules, consider and modify ongoing behavior, and form plans for future action.

Language-impaired children may have difficulty keeping up with their peers' verbal exchanges and drift to the sidelines in social situations, or they may become frustrated and "act out" or have tantrums [47].

Etiology

Social and environmental factors

In children, development of language is influenced by any factor that affects overall cognitive and social development. By 18 to 24 months of age, children who live in environments characterized by low parental education, poverty, high family and social stress, and low expressiveness are often delayed in expressive language compared with more advantaged peers [48,49]. Although children from bilingual homes may be somewhat slower in acquiring expressive language, in the absence of other adverse factors they are no more likely to be delayed by age 2 years [50]. Research on the effects of birth order on language development has been inconclusive. In a recent large community sample of children, later-born children were at greater risk for poor expressive language competence [48]. The impact of birth order effects in most research, however, has been found to be rather small [51–53]. Birth order does not seem to be a risk factor for the development of SLI [54].

Health factors

Birth defect syndromes

Delayed language development is associated with a wide range of neurologic and birth defect syndromes. The most common association is with nonspecific mental retardation, but several known syndromes have distinct language patterns. For example, as noted previously, children with Williams syndrome have fluent but pragmatically disordered language development. Children with fragile X syndrome frequently perseverate on words, phrases, and topics. Their speech is typically hard to understand because of cluttering (ie, fast, bunched together words) and mumbling [55].

Prenatal and perinatal factors

Several studies have shown that adverse prenatal and perinatal factors may contribute to poor language development. Among children born prematurely, between 20% and 40% of very low birth weight survivors have been found to have language delays as toddlers and preschoolers [56,57]. Bronchopulmonary dysplasia has recently been shown to affect the language development at age 3 years among very low birth weight infants after controlling for the effects of sociodemographic and other medical risk factors [58]. Even in less severely affected children, low birth weight (<2500 g) and 5-minute Apgar scores less than 3 have been found to increase risk for language delay [59].

Traumatic brain injury

Following severe traumatic brain injury, neurodevelopmental sequelae in children may include speech, language, and swallowing problems. Symptoms of language dysfunction may include restricted output and lack of initiation of speech, difficulty in word retrieval, pragmatic disorders in conversation, inability to comprehend figurative language, and limited verbal memory [60]. Speech sequelae may include apraxic or dysarthric impairments caused by oral motor programming deficits or weakness of the oropharyngeal musculature. In the posttraumatic period, declines in general cognitive ability may parallel decreased language competence [61,62].

Hearing disorders

With implementation of universal newborn hearing screening, most children with congenital deafness likely are identified very early in life and receive early language intervention services. Babies with significant bilateral hearing impairment who are diagnosed before the age of 6 months and receive appropriate intervention have significantly better language levels than children identified after the age of 6 months [63,64]. It is difficult to distinguish infants with severe-to-profound hearing loss and normally hearing infants until shortly after the onset of babbling. Although deaf infants babble, their vocalizations typically have fewer consonant sounds and they produce fewer multisyllabic utterances than hearing babies. The speech of children with mild-to-moderate hearing loss resembles that of normally hearing children. The former usually exhibit a delay in language development, acquiring language in a normal developmental sequence but at a slower rate than their normally developing peers. For the most part, the speech of hearing impaired children is intelligible, but sounds of low intensity, high frequency, or short duration are most commonly affected. Most speech errors include consonants and consonant blends [65]. Although unilateral hearing loss may not prevent acquisition of normal speech and language ability, sound localization and speech discrimination, especially in a noisy environment, often create problems for children in a school or social setting. All children with suspected language delays or disorders should receive audiometric evaluation as part of a complete evaluation.

The potential impact of frequent otitis media in young children with respect to speech and language development has been the subject of considerable debate and research. At present, there is no compelling evidence that a history of otitis media with effusion during preschool years is associated with clinically significant deficits in receptive or expressive language, including measures of vocabulary, syntax, or speech [66,67]. Furthermore, Paradise and colleagues [68] noted that, in young children with persistent otitis media with effusion, myringotomy with the insertion of tympanostomy tubes did not result in improved developmental outcomes by 6 years of age.

Anatomic abnormalities

Early researchers noted similarities between acquired aphasia in adults and childhood language disorder, and expected to find similar lesions in the brains of affected children. Neuroimaging studies have been unable, or inconclusive, however, in identifying brain lesions in most children with SLI. Furthermore, risk factors for neurologic injury are absent in most of these children. In a minority of children, a diverse array of anatomic abnormalities has been identified in regions of the brain that are central to language processing: white matter lesions [69]; abnormalities of white matter volume [70]; ventricular enlargement; focal gray matter heterotopia within the right and left parietotemporal white matter; abnormal morphology of the pars triangularis in the inferior frontal gyrus (part of Broca's area) [71]; reduced volume of the caudate nucleus [72]; atypical patterns of asymmetry of language cortex [73]; and increased thickness of the corpus callosum. Postmortem studies of children with language disorders have found atypical symmetry of the plana temporale and cortical dysplasia in the region of the Sylvian fissure (part of Wernicke's area). Despite these findings, specific relationships between these anatomic findings and the associated clinical features have not been established. As a result, currently available neuroimaging techniques add little useful information to standard practice in diagnosing or classifying childhood language disorder.

Genetics

Genetic factors seem to exert a major influence in the development of communication skills. The sex ratio of SLI ranges from 1.3 to 5.9:1 (male-to-female) [74]. Language disorders clearly cluster in families. In a review of 14 studies that investigated family histories of children with SLI, the median incidence of a first-degree relative with language impairment or a history of language impairment was 39% (range, 24%–77%) [75]. Bishop and coworkers [76] found the concordance rate for SLI to be 72% for monozygotic twins compared with 49% for dizygotic twins when the criteria of a 20-point discrepancy between verbal and nonverbal IQ was used. When less stringent criteria were used, the concordance rate increased to 90% in monozygotic twins and 62% in dizygotic twins.

Atypical perisylvian asymmetries and cortical atrophy have been noted in first-degree relatives of children with SLI [77]. Clarke and Plante [78] identified brain morphologic anomalies consisting of an extra sulcus in the inferior frontal gyrus of adults who had evidence of a residual language disorder. Most of these adults with this trait were parents of a language-disordered child. Even if there was no other family member with a language disorder, the morphologic anomaly was strongly associated with the adult's language abilities.

Research has identified a number of potential gene loci for language disorders, but no consistent genetic markers have been clearly established. The most plausible genetic mechanism involves a disruption in the timing of early prenatal neurogenesis affecting migration of nerve cells from the germinal matrix to the cerebral cortex. The resulting microanatomic changes produce a neural network less efficient in processing language information.

Auditory-temporal processing deficit

Interpretation of speech requires the ability to determine the spectral shape of sound, and to detect and discriminate the modulation of a wide range of sound frequencies. Additionally, this information must be processed over time to capture the extremely fast changes of consonant sounds and the longer changes of the communicative utterances. Furthermore, listeners must discriminate and interpret speech sounds even when these arrive against a background of other noises [79]. Such abilities develop very early in life, perhaps even in utero. By 6 to 8 months of age, infants can discriminate sounds from their native language in preference to nonnative or nonsense speech sounds. Tallal [80] has suggested that speech-language disorders are strongly associated with an inability to process rapidly changing information. When auditory stimuli are either brief or rapid, children with SLI have difficulty discriminating among them. When the same stimuli are lengthened or presented at a slower rate, however, performance improves [81,82]. These researchers were able to predict accurately the types of speech sounds that cause greatest difficulty. For example, vowels, which have a longer duration and little change in the levels of energy in a given frequency band, are easier to discriminate than stop consonants, characterized by a changing pattern of intensity at different frequencies. Furthermore, Tallal and colleagues [83] demonstrated that even brief steady-state stimuli were difficult to discriminate if rapidly followed by another acoustic stimulus. According to this theory, deficits in processing speed are not limited to auditory stimuli, because children with SLI have similar difficulties coping with brief or rapid events in other sensory modalities. Tallal and colleagues [83] claim that training children to process rapid auditory information improves language skills. Other researchers, however, have not replicated these findings. For example, in contrast to Tallal and colleagues' [83] theory, Bishop and colleagues [84] found that in comparing group differences between SLI children and normal controls, the processing of auditory information was greater at slower than at faster rates of presentation. Furthermore, Bishop and colleagues [85] noted that although some of the control children had difficulties in processing auditory information, they had no identified language disorder.

Phonologic short-term memory deficit

Several investigators have suggested that a core deficit in phonologic short-term memory is a core feature of SLI [11,12,86]. In both typically developing and language-impaired children, tests of phonologic short-term memory are associated with growth of receptive vocabulary over time.

One of the most powerful predictors of vocabulary is performance on a test of nonword repetition: nonwords were initially used to eliminate potential confounding that might result from an underlying deficit in word knowledge. As the number of syllables of these nonwords increases beyond four to five, children with SLI have increasing difficulty repeating them correctly, when compared with normally developing peers. Adequate short-term memory capacity permits the on-line integration of lexical, phonologic, and syntactic information that allows one to comprehend and produce language at an age-appropriate level [87,88]. In essence, one must retain the early processed components in memory store while continuing to process subsequent information. Faulty comprehension may result from slower than normal processing speed with resulting inaccurate or incomplete interpretation of the whole string. Alternatively, rapid decay of information in short-term memory may cause the initial part of a sentence to be lost before crucial, later-arriving information has been processed [89]. Whether this deficit reflects poor perception of speech sounds, faulty encoding of the information, or too rapid decay of memory, however, is not clear.

Subtle disorders of synaptic connectivity

From a diagnostic perspective, researchers have defined SLI by the presence of significant language delay or disorder in individuals who have otherwise intact nonverbal cognitive ability. This clinical picture suggests the possibility that a focal brain lesion, or "modular deficit," underlies this disorder. Most children with SLI have normal neurologic examinations, and neuroimaging studies rarely reveal focal abnormalities in brain structure. To the contrary, very young infants who experience brain damage, even to left hemisphere regions typically associated with language processing, show remarkable capacity to develop normal language function, albeit at a slower rate than control children. By middle childhood, however, few differences in language function can be identified.

Advanced computer models suggest that modular-appearing functional deficits can arise from subtle disturbances in the efficiency of highly integrated neural networks [90]. For example, by removing interconnections between processing stages, adding "noise" in the processing circuits, and altering the discriminability to the input stage of processing units, patterns resembling those seen in humans with a variety of acquired and developmental disorders can be produced. Whether the disorders in humans originate from minor structural variations or arise from differences in the interactions of neurons as they "wire up" to create functional circuits, the end result can resemble a discrete functional (modular) deficit [91].

In many ways, the neural network model goes a long way toward explaining the empirical evidence for SLI. For example, although clinicians have tried to identify distinct subtypes of language disorder, differences between them are graded rather than discrete. Observations by Tallal and others that individuals with SLI have difficulty processing preverbal auditory stimuli are consistent with subtle inefficiencies in an elementary component of a complex neural system. The association of deficient short-term memory in SLI, as evidenced by difficulty with nonword repetition tasks, is consistent with dysfunction in processing of auditory information at the phonemic level. Furthermore, processing dysfunction is not confined to auditory or linguistic information because individuals with SLI often have difficulty with a variety of fine motor and other cognitive skills. Finally, long-term follow-up suggests that the relative lack of linguistic experience has a detrimental effect on cognitive and social development. By adulthood, children with persisting severe language impairments gradually resemble those who started life with more obvious cognitive and social disabilities. Persistence of less efficient processing methods may help to explain why adults who seem to have recovered from SLI often still perform poorly when challenged with a high verbal information load, or when they are required to deal with novel information [92].

Prognosis

Language outcomes

Although it is very difficult to predict accurately the functional language outcome of individual children who present with delayed onset of talking, longitudinal research provides some guidance regarding prognosis. Nonverbal intelligence is among the most important variables determining outcome of early speech-language delay. Additionally, the course of language development is also strongly associated with long-term outcome: improvement in language ability is associated with better prognosis.

Language impairments in preschool children that are confined to expressive phonology are associated with low risk of later language or reading problems. In most children, phonologically based articulation problems resolve by the time of school entry [23,93,94]. Catts [95] noted little correlation between articulation ability in kindergarten and reading ability in first and second grade. Children who lack phonologic awareness of words (eg, who cannot complete rhymes or identify phoneme sounds in words), however, are at risk for later reading problems in word recognition [96].

Bishop and Edmundson [23] followed 87 middle-class, preschool-age speech-language-impaired children, who had been classified as having either normal nonverbal intelligence (SLI) or retarded nonverbal intelligence (ie, at least 2 SD below the mean). Children with hearing impairments and autism were not included in their sample. Eighteen months later, at mean age 5 years 6 months, 37% had resolved their language impairment. Among children with normal nonverbal intelligence (SLI group), 44% had achieved normal language skills, whereas 89% of the children with retarded nonverbal intelligence continued to show language delays. At ages 15 to 16 years,

71 of the original cohort of children who had been evaluated at age 4 years were re-examined [97].

These subjects were compared with normally developing children from the same social class and geographic background. The results indicated that the children whose early language impairments had improved by age 5.5 years had slightly lower, but not statistically significant, scores on tests of expressive and receptive vocabulary, picture naming, and receptive grammar compared with controls. Significant deficits were noted, however, on tasks that tapped short-term verbal memory (ie, sentence repetition) and phonologic skills (ie, nonword repetition and "spoonerism" tasks). The nonverbal intellectual abilities of this group were indistinguishable from the controls. Their reading skills were significantly poorer than the control group's; however, they were generally consistent with predictions based on intellectual scores, and they were not considered dyslexic by standard definition.

The long-term prognosis for children with persisting language deficits at age 5.5 years was generally very poor. Eighty percent of the SLI group (ie, with normal nonverbal intellectual scores) had verbal composite scores more than 1 SD below the mean, and 37% scored more than 2 SD below the mean. As a group, receptive and expressive language performance of the SLI group was indistinguishable from those who were generally delayed (in language and nonverbal intelligence) at 5.5 years. Most striking, however, was the finding that almost half (47%) of the persistent SLI group's nonverbal composite scores were more than 1 SD below the mean, and 20% were more than 2 SD below the mean. Among the children who were impaired in both verbal and nonverbal abilities, 60% had verbal composite scores and 47% had nonverbal composite scores more than 2 SD below the mean.

Bishop and Edmondsons's [23] results strongly suggest that there is little likelihood of children outgrowing their language difficulties beyond age 5 years. Specifically, children whose language impairments did not improve by the time of school entry were at very high risk of continued language, literacy, and educational difficulties throughout childhood and adolescent years. Although those children whose early language delays seemed to resolve by age 5 had a good prognosis for spoken language development, their phonologic skills remained weak and they experienced difficulty in reading ability compared with normally developing peers.

Tomblin and colleagues [92] followed up a group of 35 young adults who had been evaluated at around 8 years old and had received the diagnosis of SLI. These individuals were compared with 35 normally developing high school and college students. The results were consistent with the findings of Bishop and colleagues [24] that residual language processing deficits were identifiable in early adulthood. A battery of four measures correctly identified the early language-impaired from normally developing individuals with an error rate of only 3%. These measures included the Modified Token

Test (comprehension of sentences); the Peabody Picture Vocabulary Test-Revised (receptive vocabulary); the Written Spelling test of the Multilingual Aphasia Examination; and the Boston Naming Test (word retrieval).

Beitchman and colleagues [98,99] examined 1655 5-year-old children in a community-based sample and identified 315 who failed a speech and language screening protocol. From a population sample of 1655 children, 315 failed a speech and language screening protocol. Of these, 142 were evaluated further, and each child was matched with a normally developing child and followed over time. Seven years later, at chronologic age 12 years, children who had pervasive language difficulties at age 5 years continued to have poor language skills and lower academic achievement compared with normally developing children or those with just poor articulation skills at baseline.

Clegg and colleagues [100] reported the longest sequential follow-up study of normally intelligent but severely language-impaired children. Persisting language difficulty was associated with very poor global developmental outcome, and limited social adjustment in adulthood. As originally designed, the study involved a longitudinal comparison of language-impaired children with relatively high-functioning autistic children. The study sample consisted of children who were recruited from special hospital and school programs in the United Kingdom that specialized in treating children with severe language disorders or autism [101]. The language-impaired group consisted of 23 boys, between the ages of 4 and 9 years, who had severe delays in expressive and receptive language but did not show evidence of clear autistic features. All had a performance IQ of at least 70, and no specific medical etiology was established for the language impairment. They were re-examined at 13 years, 24 years, and 36 years of age and compared with a normally developing sibling and an IQ-matched peer using a variety of cognitive, language, academic, and social-emotional measures. Not surprisingly, those with persisting severe language impairment had the poorest outcomes in all areas. Overall, the language-disordered individuals' verbal and performance IQ were on average 2 SD below that of their siblings. Academically, the language-impaired individuals achieved a reading level equivalent of only 10 years. Only one individual attained a Certificate of Secondary Education. In their mid-thirties, only 59% of the language-impaired individuals were employed. Furthermore, their employment histories were unstable and almost two thirds had experienced prolonged periods of unemployment exceeding 2 years. This pattern compared with a 94% employment rate for their siblings. The types of employment of the language-impaired adults included unskilled and manual labor occupations.

Nineteen boys were initially diagnosed as having autism using criteria available in the 1960s [102]. For the most part, the autistic children showed improvement in language ability over time. As expected, their social skills remained very poor. In contrast, the language-impaired children showed a variable outcome over time. There was a steady decline in cognitive and social skills, however, among the language-impaired children as they aged. By age 23 years, although the language-impaired group was generally more functional, there was great overlap between the two groups in terms of reading, spelling, and writing skills. Among those originally diagnosed with language impairment, half continued to have problems sustaining a conversation, 40% had some difficulties in the spontaneous reporting of events, one quarter were said to have immature syntax, and half showed some prosodic oddities. Equally striking was the finding that nearly a third of the individuals in the language-impaired group had interests that occupied an unusual amount of time. For example, five were "unusually routinized" and four had unusually negative reactions to change; two had very definite preoccupations that took up almost all of their free time and intruded into family life. More than half had some problems establishing spontaneous, reciprocal relationships; more than a third had no particular friends, and two thirds had not developed a close relationship with the opposite sex. Most still lived at home with their parents, and leisure activities were often restricted. Employment levels were low, with jobs often being temporary or poorly paid.

The authors noted that the tendency toward convergence in adulthood of symptoms that initially seem more distinct suggests a stronger commonality between autism and language disorders than is usually thought. This is also in keeping with the observation that relatives of autistic probands often have language disorders and other atypical symptoms (the so-called "broader autism phenotype") [103–105].

Of note is the fact that in all of the longitudinal studies substantial declines were observed in nonverbal cognitive abilities, particularly in children who did not show significant resolution of language impairment during middle school years. Although the specific reasons for this phenomenon are not clear, it may represent a failure of the normal "bootstrapping" effect of language skills on general cognitive development, in which the acquisition of increasingly abstract concepts is impaired [106].

Behavioral and social outcomes

In the Beitchman and colleagues [107] study, early language disorder was also associated with poor emotional, behavioral, and social outcome 7 and 14 years later. Young adults with early language impairment had significantly elevated rates of anxiety disorders (27%) compared with speech-impaired only (15.8%) and with typically developing controls (8.1%). Not surprisingly, given these individuals' problems associated with speaking to others and their difficulty in managing social interactions, social phobia was the most common type of anxiety disorder noted. This group also exhibited an increased rate of antisocial behavior (19.5%) compared with speech-impaired only (13.2%) and with typically developing controls (7.8%). After controlling for the effects of verbal IQ, demographic, and family variables, a significant association was found, primarily in boys, between delinquency symptoms and early language impairment.

Vallance and colleagues [108] explored in depth the association between language impairment and psychiatric disorder. Children referred for psychiatric care without language impairment were noted to be less fluent and efficient in speech, and to use less emotional language than nonpsychiatrically referred children and nonreferred controls. Despite these differences, however, they were able to produce linguistically rich, cohesive, and coherent narratives. The language pattern of psychiatrically referred children with language impairments was characterized by a greater reliance on simple, short sentences, and poor cohesion within and across sentences. As a result, these children were more likely to describe events rather than explain the reasons for peoples' actions and outcomes of events. Language-impaired children seem to be at a disadvantage because disruptions in the ability to use language limit their ability to obtain meaning from their social context.

In the Clegg and colleagues [100] study noted previously, only 40% of the language-impaired adults were living independently, compared with nearly all of their siblings. Nearly half of the language-impaired adults had sustained problems in establishing relationships across acquaintances, friendships, and sexual relationships. They tended to live socially restricted lives that affected their opportunities for employment and independent living. Most surprising was the absence of psychiatric disorders that might be attributable to their communication and social impairments.

Clinical case histories

Case 1 (apraxia)

JZ, a 3-year-, 7-month-old boy, was not yet saying any words. He could use several signs and some Picture Exchange Communication System cards. He made the sound "mama" indiscriminately and often vocalized while pointing things out to his parents. He was clearly frustrated when parents did not understand what he was trying to say.

JZ clearly recognized letters of the alphabet, and selectively pointed them out for others to pronounce for him. Both his parents, and the teachers at his early childhood program, noted that JZ seemed to understand a lot of what was said around him. He could follow single-step commands and look for named objects that were located in a different room of the house. He tried to interact with other children, and they enjoyed being with him. He had no difficulty adapting to new settings.

He was helpful around the house, and wanted his parents to be involved in his activities. He pretended he was flying his toy airplane and he enjoyed playing with action figures.

JZ was the product of a normal pregnancy, labor, and delivery. His past medical history was unremarkable. In the first few months of life, JZ had difficulty nursing, and his weight gain was poor despite switching to a bottle. He smiled at 1 to 2 months, sat up at 5 months, and walked independently at 9 months. Mother recalled that he waved "bye-bye" at 9 months. He was very quiet as an infant and did not start to babble until he was almost 2 years old. Formal hearing testing was done in infancy and was normal. A review of the family history revealed that mother received speech therapy as a child for an articulation problem. She also had symptoms of dyslexia. No other family members had difficulty with speech, language, learning, or general development as children.

Physical examination was normal, with the exception of generalized hypotonia and increased range of motion of the joints. Oral motor functions were intact. Cognitive assessment, using the Merrill-Palmer Revised Scales of Development (a nonverbal measure), found JZ to function in the borderline range (standard score, 74). On the Preschool Language Scale, his receptive and expressive language skills were mildly-to-moderately delayed. His auditory comprehension standard score was 57 and expressive communication standard score was 50. The speech pathologist noted that JZ had a limited expressive vocabulary and experienced significant difficulty with verbal imitation tasks. His range of speech sounds was severely restricted and he rarely used combinations of consonants and vowels. No true words were heard during the evaluation session. Despite his verbal difficulties, JZ was observed to request that all adults sign the name of objects with him. The psychologist noted:

> He would indicate this request by walking over to each adult, demonstrating the sign continuously while looking at them until they produced the sign. Once produced, he would move on to the next adult. After all adults had completed the activity, he would appear content and move on to another activity. On one occasion, he initiated stacking hands on top of each other with one of the family members. He then insisted that all adults join in and stack their hands on the pile. Once this was completed, JZ smiled at all the adults and then allowed them to return to their seats.

JZ was diagnosed with apraxia of speech. Additional concerns included possible delay-disorder in receptive language ability and borderline cognitive ability.

One year later, at 4 years 10 months, JZ returned for evaluation. His parents reported that he had learned to say parts of words (eg, he would say "e-e-e" for cookie). He used more than 30 signs, singly and in combination, and he said "yes" and "no" clearly. He could say most of the letters of the alphabet, and would spell his name aloud. According to his parents, JZ's frustration level decreased as his ability to communicate orally increased. Repeat cognitive testing using the Preschool Performance Scale found his nonverbal abilities to be in the solid average range (IQ 98). Expressive skills were below a 3-year level, however, whereas receptive skills were at a 4-year 6-month level.

Case 2 (specific language impairment)

KB was seen for a multidisciplinary evaluation for delayed language development when he was 23 months old. At 18 months of age, he did not use any recognizable words. After several months of Birth to Three services he was able use several signs properly. He also seemed to understand a few simple verbal commands. There were no concerns about his social skills and he was observed to interact well with other children. KB pointed to pictures in books and used question-like inflected jargon while turning to his parents. He understood the function of common objects and combined toys in play. Parents had no concerns about his general health. The family history was significant. Both parents had a history of depression and father was treated for attention-deficit/hyperactivity disorder as a child. KB's 6-year-old brother was receiving special education services for a language disorder. Mother's pregnancy with KB was normal, and the birth and postnatal medical history were unremarkable.

The initial evaluations found KB's receptive and expressive skills to be mildly delayed, whereas nonverbal cognitive measures were at age level. Physical and neurologic examinations were normal. A mixed expressive and receptive language disorder was suspected. The parents were encouraged to continue the early intervention program and a follow-up developmental assessment was scheduled in 1 year.

Over the next few years, KB returned for annual re-evaluations. When seen at 4 years old, his nonverbal IQ was 97 and he demonstrated evidence of pretend play, imitation, and joint referencing behaviors. His language skills had improved dramatically, but he was still delayed for his age. Spontaneous communication included echolalia and perseveration on movie themes. He was also able to express his feelings and to "negotiate" with his older brother. KB continued to show improvement in his overall communication ability and he continued to receive speech therapy services in the public school system. At age 7 years, KB was able to recognize many sight words and he was beginning to analyze phonetically unfamiliar words. He was able to hold a conversation, but he struggled with time concepts, pronouns, and gender references. He socialized well with peers, but became frustrated easily and would break down crying if he did not understand what the others were doing. KB's teachers raised a concern about symptoms of attention-deficit/hyperactivity disorder and his primary care pediatrician started a stimulant medication with some success.

When seen again at age 11 years, KB was in a regular fourth grade class with no speech therapy or special education support services. His intellectual abilities remained in the average range and his academic skills were at grade level in all subjects. Assessment of language abilities identified persisting difficulty with understanding and use of complex grammar and verbal memory. The speech pathologist noted that he revised his statements repeatedly to formulate "correct" sentences. Some residual pragmatic conversational weaknesses were also observed. Eye contact was not always maintained with his conversational partner, he did not often signal when changing topics, and his use of idioms and metaphors was inappropriate. Parents also expressed concern about escalating behavior problems. Although he continued to take the stimulant medication, he was having angry outbursts in school. Both parents and teachers observed him to be very anxious with change in routines and he seemed to be easily frustrated. KB expressed frequent feelings of sadness. After each emotional episode, he expressed remorse. A selective serotonin reuptake inhibitor medication was started with minimal improvement in his symptoms. Over the next several months, the emotional outbursts escalated and he was referred to a child psychiatrist for treatment of a mood disorder.

Summary

Acquisition of functional communication ability is an essential part of human development. Delays and disorders of language comprehension or expression are very common in children and are frequently associated with a wide range of cognitive, academic, social, and emotional dysfunctions. Children's language development should be assessed at each encounter with a pediatric health care provider. Familiarization with the various clinical patterns fosters early identification and treatment of communication disorders. Although the prognosis for most children with early speech and language delay is generally favorable, a significant proportion of children with persistent disorders of communication experience increasing challenges over time. These children should be followed closely and the health care provider must be alert to the emergence of symptoms of emotional and behavioral disorders, learning disabilities, and social maladjustment. At present, diagnosis of communication disorders is largely based on clinical features. In the future, emerging neuroimaging and genetic technologies may allow more objective diagnosis and prognosis of language disorders.

References

[1] Pinker S. The language instinct. New York: William Morrow and Co, Inc.; 1994. p. 18, 52.
[2] Rescorla L. The language development survey: a screening tool for delayed language in toddlers. J Speech Hear Disord 1989;54:587–99.
[3] Stevenson J, Richman N. The prevalence of language delay in a population of three-year-old children and its association with general retardation. Dev Med Child Neurol 1976;18: 431–41.
[4] Tomblin JB, Records HL, Buckwater P, et al. Prevalence of specific language impairment in kindergarten children. J Speech Lang Hear Res 1997;40:1245–60.
[5] Rapin I, Allen D. Developmental language disorders: nosologic considerations. In: Kirk U, editor. Neuropsychology of language, reading, and spelling. New York: Academic Press; 1983.
[6] American Psychiatric Association. Diagnostic and statistical manual of mental disorders. 4th edition. Washington, DC: American Psychiatric Association; 1994.

[7] Leonard LB. Children with specific language impairment. Cambridge (MA): the MIT Press; 1998.

[8] Tomblin JB, Records NL, Zhang X. A system for the diagnosis of specific language impairment in kindergarten children. J Speech Lang Hear Res 1996;39:1284–94.

[9] Miller JF, Chapman RS, MacKenzie H. Individual difference in the language acquisition patterns of mentally retarded children. Proceedings of the Symposium on Research in Child Language Disorders 1981;2:130–46.

[10] Bishop DVM. Uncommon understanding: development and disorders of language comprehension in children. East Sussex (UK): Psychology Press Limited; 1997. p. 20, 143, 147.

[11] Bishop DVM, North T, Donlan C. Nonword repetition as a behavioural marker for inherited language impairment: evidence from a twin study. J Child Psychol Psychiatry 1996;37:391–403.

[12] Gathercole SE, Baddeley AD. Phonological memory deficits in language disordered children: is there a causal connection? J Mem Lang 1990;29:336–60.

[13] Botting N, Conti-Ramsden G. Non-word repetition and language development in children with specific language impairment (SLI). Int J Lang Commun Disord 2001;36:421–32.

[14] Van der Lely HKJ, Stollwerck L. A grammatical specific language impairment in children: an autosomal dominant inheritance? Brain Lang 1996;52:484–504.

[15] Van der Lely HKJ, Rosen S, McClelland A. Evidence for a grammar-specific deficit in children. Curr Biol 1998;8:1253–8.

[16] Lazaar RT, Warr-Leeper GA, Nicholson CB, et al. Elementary school teachers' use of multiple meaning expressions. Lang Speech Hear Serv Sch 1989;20:240–50.

[17] Rinaldi W. Pragmatic comprehension in secondary school-aged students with specific developmental language disorder. Int J Lang Commun Disord 2000;35:1–29.

[18] Shriberg LD, Kwiatkowski J. Developmental phonological disorders I: a clinical profile. J Speech Hear Res 1994;37:1100–26.

[19] Johnson C, Beitchman JH. Phonological disorders. In: Sadock BJ, Sadock VA, editors. Kaplan and Sadock's comprehensive textbook of psychiatry. 7th edition. Baltimore (MD): Lippincott Williams and Wilkins; 1999. p. 2945–60.

[20] Ferry PC, Hall SM, Hicks JL. Dilapidated speech: developmental verbal dyspraxia. Dev Med Child Neurol 1975;17:749–56.

[21] Velleman SL, Strand K. Developmental verbal dyspraxia. In: Bernthal JE, Bankson NW, editors. Child phonology: characteristics, assessment, and intervention with special populations. New York: Thieme; 1994. p. 110–39.

[22] Lewis BA, Freebairn LA, Hansen A, et al. Family pedigrees of children with suspected childhood apraxia of speech. J Commun Disord 2004;37:157–75.

[23] Bishop DVM, Edmundson A. Language-impaired 4-year-olds: distinguishing transient from persistent impairment. J Speech Hear Disord 1987;52:156–73.

[24] Paul R, Smith R. Narrative skills in 4-year-olds with normal, impaired, and late-developing language. J Speech Hear Res 1993;36:592–8.

[25] Sowell T. The Einstein syndrome: bright children who talk late. New York: Basic Books; 2001.

[26] Stein MT, Parker S, Coplan J, et al. Expressive language delay in a toddler. J Dev Behav Pediatr 2001;22(2 Suppl):S99–103.

[27] Weismer SE, Murray-Branch J, Miller JF. A prospective longitudinal study of language development in late talkers. J Speech Hear Res 1994;37:852–67.

[28] Webster RI, Majnemer A, Platt RW, et al. Motor function at school age in children with a preschool diagnosis of developmental language impairment. J Pediatr 2005;146:80–5.

[29] Powell RP, Bishop DV. Clumsiness and perceptual problems in children with specific language impairment. Dev Med Child Neurol 1992;34:755–65.

[30] Bishop DVM. Motor immaturity and specific speech and language impairment: evidence for a common genetic basis. Am J Med Genet 2002;114:56–63.

[31] Hill E. A dyspraxic deficit in specific language impairment and developmental coordination disorder? Evidence from hand and arm movements. Dev Med Child Neurol 1998;40: 388–95.

[32] Nelson LK, Kamhi AG, Apel K. Cognitive strengths and weaknesses in language-impaired children: one more look. J Speech Hear Disord 1987;52:30–6.

[33] Rapin I. Preschool children with inadequate communication. London: Mac Keith Press; 1996.

[34] Hick R, Botting N, Conti-Ramsden G. Cognitive abilities in children with specific language impairment: consideration of visuo-spatial skills. Int J Lang Commun Disord 2005;40: 137–49.

[35] Bavin EL, Wilson PH, Maruff P, et al. Spatio-visual memory of children with specific language impairment: evidence for generalized processing problems. Int J Lang Commun Disord 2005;40:319–32.

[36] Ors M. Time to drop "specific" in "specific language impairment". Acta Paediatr 2002;91: 1025–6.

[37] Fernell E, Norrelgen F, Bozkurt I, et al. Developmental profiles and auditory perception in 25 children attending special preschools for language-impaired children. Acta Paediatr 2002;91:1108–15.

[38] Beitchman JH, Nair R, Clegg M, et al. Prevalence of psychiatric disorders in children with speech and language disorders. J Am Acad Child Adolesc Psychiatry 1986;25: 528–35.

[39] Gualtieri T, Koriath U, Van Bourgondien M, et al. Language disorders in children referred for psychiatric services. J Am Acad Child Adolesc Psychiatry 1983;22:165–71.

[40] Silva PA, Williams S, McGee R. A longitudinal study of children with developmental language delay at age three: later intelligence, reading and behaviour problems. Dev Med Child Neurol 1987;29:630–40.

[41] Beitchman JH, Cohen JN, Konstantareas MM, et al, editors. Language, learning, and behavior disorders: developmental, biological, and clinical perspectives. New York: Cambridge University Press; 1996.

[42] Cantwell DP, Baker L. Psychiatric and developmental disorders in children with communication disorders. Washington, DC: American Psychiatric Press; 1991.

[43] Beitchman JH, Hood J, Rochon J, et al. Empirical classification of speech/language impairment in children: II. Behavioral characteristics. J Am Acad Child Adolesc Psychiatry 1989; 28:118–23.

[44] Cohen NJ, Davine M, Horodezky N, et al. Unsuspected language impairment in psychiatrically disturbed children: prevalence and language and behavioral characteristics. J Am Acad Child Adolesc Psychiatry 1993;32:595–603.

[45] Cohen N, Horodezky NB. Language impairments and psychopathology. J Am Acad Child Adolesc Psychiatry 1998;37:461–2.

[46] Berk LE. Children's private speech. In: Berk LE, Diaz RM, editors. Private speech: from social interaction to self-regulation. Hillsdale (NJ): Erlbaum; 1992. p. 17–53.

[47] Brownlie EB, Beitchman JH, Escobar M, et al. Early language impairment and young adult delinquent and aggressive behavior. J Abnorm Child Psychol 2004;32:453–67.

[48] Horwitz SM, Irwin JR, Briggs-Gowan MJ, et al. Language delay in a community cohort of young children. J Am Acad Child Adolesc Psychiatry 2003;42:932–40.

[49] King TM, Rosenberg LA, Fuddy L, et al. Prevalence and early identification of language delays among at-risk three year olds. J Dev Behav Pediatr 2005;26:293–303.

[50] Patterson J. What bilingual toddlers hear and say: language input and word combinations. Communication Disord Q 1999;21:32–8.

[51] Bornstein MH, Leach DB, Haynes OM. Vocabulary competence in first- and second born siblings of the same chronological age. J Child Lang 2004;31:855–73.

[52] Pine JM. Variation in vocabulary development as a function of birth order. Child Dev 1995; 66:272–81.

[53] Fenson L, Dale PS, Reznick JS, et al. Variability in early communicative development. Monogr Soc Res Child Dev 1994;59:1–173.

[54] Tomblin JB. The effect of birth order on the occurrence of developmental language impairment. Br J Disord Commun 1990;25:77–84.

[55] Hanson DM, Jackson AW, Hagerman RJ. Speech disturbances (cluttering) in mildly impaired males with the Martin-Bell/fragile X syndrome. Am J Med Genet 1986;7: 471–89.

[56] Aram D, Hack M, Hawkins S, et al. Very low birthweight children and speech and language development. J Speech Hear Res 1991;34:1169–79.

[57] Weisglas-Kuperus N, Baerts W, DeGraff MA, et al. Hearing and language in preschool very low birthweight children. Int J Pediatr Otorhinolaryngol 1993;26:129–40.

[58] Singer LT, Siegel AC, Lewis B, et al. Preschool language outcomes of children with history of bronchopulmonary dysplasia and very low birth weight. J Dev Behav Pediatr 2001;22: 19–26.

[59] Stanton-Chapman TL, Chapman DA, Bainbridge NL, et al. Identification of early risk factors for language impairment. Res Dev Disabil 2002;23:390–405.

[60] Ylvisaker M. Communication outcome following traumatic brain injury. Semin Speech Lang 1992;13:239–50.

[61] Jordan FM, Ashton R. Language performance of severely closed head injured children. Brain Inj 1996;10:91–8.

[62] Jordan FM, Cremona Meteyard S, King A. High-level linguistic disturbances subsequent to childhood closed head injury. Brain Inj 1996;10:729–38.

[63] Yoshinaga-Itano C, Sedey AL, Coulter DK, et al. Language of early- and later-identified children with hearing loss. Pediatrics 1998;102:1161–71.

[64] Moeller MP. Early intervention and language development in children who are deaf and hard of hearing. Pediatrics 2000;106(3). Available at: http://www.pediatrics.org/cgi/content/full/106/3/e43. Accessed March 29, 2007.

[65] Rigo TG. Habilitation and communication development in hearing-impaired infants and toddlers. In: Billeaud FP, editor. Communication disorders in infants and toddlers: assessment and intervention. 2nd edition. Boston: Butterworth-Heinemann; 1998. p. 179–96.

[66] Roberts JE, Rosenfeld RM, Zeisel SA. Otitis media and speech and language: a meta-analysis of prospective studies. Pediatrics 2004;113(3). Available at: http://www.pediatrics.org/cgi/content/full/113/3/e238. Accessed March 29, 2007.

[67] Paradise JL, Dollaghan CA, Campbell TF, et al. Language, speech sound production, and cognition in three-year-old children in relation to otitis media in their first three years of life. Pediatrics 2000;105:1119–30.

[68] Paradise JL, Campbell TF, Dollaghan CA, et al. Developmental outcomes after early or delayed insertion of tympanostomy tubes. N Engl J Med 2005;353:576–86.

[69] Trauner D, Wulfeck B, Tallal P, et al. Neurological and MRI profiles of children with developmental language impairment. Dev Med Child Neurol 2000;42:470–5.

[70] Herbert MR, Ziegler DA, Makris N, et al. Localization of white matter volume increase in autism and developmental language disorder. Ann Neurol 2004;55:530–40.

[71] Gauger LM, Lombardino LJ, Leonard CM. Brain morphology in children with specific language impairment. J Speech Lang Hear Res 1997;40:1272–84.

[72] Jernigan TL, Hesselink JR, Sowell E, et al. Cerebral structure on magnetic resonance imaging in language- and learning-impaired children. Arch Neurol 1991;48:539–45.

[73] Plante E, Swisher L, Vance R, et al. MRI findings in boys with specific language impairment. Brain Lang 1991;41:67–80.

[74] Tallal P, Ross R, Curtiss S. Unexpected sex ratios in families of language/learning impaired children. Neuropsychologia 1989;27:987–98.

[75] Stromswold K. Genetics of spoken language disorders. Hum Biol 1998;2:297–324.

[76] Bishop DVM, North T, Dolan C. Genetic basis of specific language impairment: evidence from a twin study. Dev Med Child Neurol 1995;37:56–71.

[77] Jackson T, Plante E. Gyral morphology in the posterior Sylvian region in families affected by developmental language disorder. Neuropsychol Rev 1996;6:81–94.

[78] Clark MM, Plante E. Morphology of the inferior frontal gyrus in developmentally language-disordered adults. Brain Lang 1998;61:288–303.

[79] Bailey PJ, Snowling MJ. Auditory processing and the development of language and literacy. Br Med Bull 2002;63:135–46.

[80] Tallal P. Rapid auditory processing in normal and disordered language development. J Speech Hear Res 1976;19:561–71.

[81] Tallal P, Piercy M. Defects of non-verbal auditory perception in children with developmental aphasia. Nature 1973;241:468–9.

[82] Tallal P, Piercy M. Developmental aphasia: impaired rate of nonverbal processing as a function of sensory modality. Neuropsychologia 1973;11:389–98.

[83] Tallal P, Miller SL, Bedi G, et al. Language comprehension in language-learning impaired children improved with acoustically modified speech. Science 1996;271:81–4.

[84] Bishop DVM, Bishop SJ, Bright P, et al. Different origin of auditory and phonological processing problems in children with language impairment: evidence from a twin study. J Speech Lang Hear Res 1999;42:155–68.

[85] Bishop DVM, Carlyon RP, Deeks JM, et al. Auditory temporal processing impairment: neither necessary nor sufficient for causing language impairment in children. J Speech Lang Hear Res 1999;42:1295–310.

[86] Montgomery JW. Sentence comprehension in children with specific language impairment: the role of phonological working memory. J Speech Hear Res 1995;38:189–99.

[87] Rice M, Wexler K, Cleave P. Specific language impairment as a period of extended optional infinitive. J Speech Hear Res 1995;38:850–63.

[88] Ellis Weismer S. Constructive comprehension abilities exhibited by language-disordered children. J Speech Hear Res 1985;28:175–84.

[89] Deevy P, Leonard LB. The comprehension of Wh- questions in children with specific language impairment. J Speech Lang Hear Res 2004;47:802–15.

[90] Thomas M, Karmiloff-Smith A. Are developmental disorders like cases of adult brain damage? Implications from connectionist modeling. Behav Brain Sci 2002;25:727–88.

[91] Morton JB, Munakata Y. What's the difference? Contrasting modular and neural network approaches to understanding developmental variability. J Dev Behav Pediatr 2005;26: 128–39.

[92] Tomblin JB, Freese PR, Records NL. Diagnosing specific language impairment in adults for the purpose of pedigree analysis. J Speech Hear Res 1992;35:832–43.

[93] Whitehurst GJ, Fischel JE. Practitioner review: early developmental language delay: what, if anything, should the clinician do about it? J Child Psychol Psychiatry 1994; 35:613–48.

[94] Bishop DVM, Adams C. A prospective study of the relationship between specific language impairment, phonological disorders and reading retardation. J Child Psychol Psychiatry 1990;31:1027–50.

[95] Catts HW. The relationship between speech-language impairments and reading disabilities. J Speech Hear Res 1993;36:948–58.

[96] Grizzle KL, Simms MD. Early language development and language learning disabilities. Pediatr Rev 2005;26:274–83.

[97] Stothard SE, Snowling MJ, Bishop DVM, et al. Language-impaired preschoolers: a follow-up into adolescence. J Speech Lang Hear Res 1998;41:407–18.

[98] Beitchman JH, Wilson B, Brownlie EB, et al. Long-term consistency in speech/language profiles: I. Developmental and academic outcomes. J Am Acad Child Adolesc Psychiatry 1996;35:804–14.

[99] Beitchman JH, Wilson B, Brownlie EB, et al. Long-term consistency in speech/language profiles: II. Behavioral, emotional, and social outcomes. J Am Acad Child Adolesc Psychiatry 1996;35:815–25.

[100] Clegg J, Hollis C, Mawhood L, et al. Developmental language disorder-a follow-up in later adult life: cognitive, language and psychosocial outcomes. J Child Psychol Psychiatry 2005; 46:128–49.
[101] Bartak L, Rutter M, Cox A. A comparative study of infantile autism and specific developmental receptive language disorders. I. The children. Br J Psychiatry 1975;126:127–45.
[102] Rutter M. Autistic children: infancy to adulthood. Semin Psychiatry 1970;2:435–50.
[103] Szatmari P, MacLean JE, Jones MB, et al. The familial aggregation of the lesser variant in biological and nonbiological relatives of PDD probands: a family history study. J Child Psychol Psychiatry 2000;41:579–86.
[104] Piven J, Palmer P, Jacobi D, et al. Broader autism phenotype: evidence from a family history study of multiple-incidence autism families. Am J Psychiatry 1997;154:185–90.
[105] Szatmari P, Jones MB, Fisman S, et al. Parents and collateral relatives of children with pervasive developmental disorder: a family history study. Am J Med Genet 1995;60:282–9.
[106] Botting N. Non-verbal cognitive development and language impairment. J Child Psychol Psychiatry 2005;46:317–26.
[107] Beitchman JH, Wilson B, Johnson CJ, et al. Fourteen-year follow-up of speech/language-impaired and control children: psychiatric outcome. J Am Acad Child Adolesc Psychiatry 2001;40:75–82.
[108] Vallance DD, Im N, Cohen NJ. Discourse deficits associated with psychiatric disorders and with language impairments in children. J Child Psychol Psychiatry 1999;40:693–704.

ELSEVIER
SAUNDERS

PEDIATRIC CLINICS
OF NORTH AMERICA

Pediatr Clin N Am 54 (2007) 469–481

Language Disorders: Autism and Other Pervasive Developmental Disorders

Helen Tager-Flusberg, PhD[a],*,
Elizabeth Caronna, MD[b]

[a]Department of Anatomy and Neurobiology, Boston University School of Medicine,
715 Albany Street, L-814, Boston, MA 02118, USA
[b]Division of Developmental and Behavioral Pediatrics, Boston Medical Center,
91 East Concord St., Maternity 5, Boston, MA 02118, USA

Autism spectrum disorders (ASD) are increasingly common neurodevelopmental disorders that encompass a range of clinical presentations characterized by functional impairments in a triad of symptoms: (1) limited reciprocal social interactions, (2) disordered verbal and nonverbal communication, and (3) restricted, repetitive behaviors or circumscribed interests [1]. Included under the umbrella of the autism spectrum are the disorders defined in the *Diagnostic and Statistical Manual of Mental Disorders, fourth edition, text revised* (*DSM-IV TR*) as pervasive developmental disorders (PDD): autistic disorder, Asperger's disorder, and pervasive developmental disorder, not otherwise specified (PDD-NOS). Rett's disorder and childhood disintegrative disorder also appear in the *DSM* classification under the rubric of PDD, but they usually are considered to be distinct from the autism spectrum. The terminology used for ASD can be confusing, because clinicians and families may use different terms to describe the same clinical entities, often using the terms "autism," "autism spectrum disorder," and "PDD" interchangeably. In this article, the term "ASD" is used to include autistic disorder, Asperger's disorder, and PDD-NOS.

Young children who have autistic disorder generally exhibit marked impairments in all three domains of the triad before the age of 3 years. Often these children are referred for evaluation around the age of 2 years because of language delay, lack of interest in social contact with children or adults, and atypical, perseverative play (eg, focusing on spinning wheels, flashing lights, or non-toy objects such as pieces of thread), although there is

---

* Corresponding author.
E-mail address: htagerf@bu.edu (H. Tager-Flusberg).

0031-3955/07/$ - see front matter © 2007 Elsevier Inc. All rights reserved.
doi:10.1016/j.pcl.2007.02.011   *pediatric.theclinics.com*

significant variability in the specific symptoms and degree of severity. Language abilities may range from being nonverbal to developing language that is highly idiosyncratic with echolalia, scripted speech, and unusual prosody (tone or inflection). At least half of all children who have autism have mental retardation; those who do not have nonverbal cognitive delays are considered to be high functioning even though they may have significant impairments in adaptive functioning and language or communication.

Much less common than the other forms of ASD, Asperger's disorder is sometimes incorrectly thought of as a mild form of autism. The degree of functional impairment in social interactions of affected individuals is variable but may be quite profound [2]. The diagnostic category itself has been controversial, and experts disagree on whether it should be considered a distinct disorder from autism [3]. As defined in *DSM-IV-TR* [4], early language development in Asperger's disorder is not delayed, (although the *DSM*'s definition of normal language development of "single words used by age 2 years, communicative phrases used by age 3 years" would, in general, be considered moderately delayed), and intellectual abilities are at least average but can be superior. Social interactions, including use of eye gaze and body postures, development of friendships, and social reciprocity, are atypical. Intense, restricted, or all-encompassing interests are common and may be developmentally appropriate in content (eg, dinosaurs) or quite unusual (eg, the intricacies of a municipal recycling program). Most children who have Asperger's disorder are not identified until early school age, when social difficulties with other children become impossible to ignore or to explain away as mere quirkiness. Language skills, including articulation, vocabulary, and grammatical abilities, may be preserved, although social or pragmatic aspects of language, such as the ability to engage in the give-and-take of social discourse, are impaired [5]. These children have been described as "little professors" who may use advanced vocabulary, speak in monologues or with a pedantic style, have difficulty with abstract or nonliteral language, and have unusual prosody [6–8].

PDD-NOS is a term for individuals who show symptoms of ASD but do not meet full *DSM* criteria for autistic disorder or Asperger's disorder because of atypical or subthreshold symptoms or later age of onset. Changes in the text revision of *DSM-IV* specified that this diagnosis is reserved for individuals with, at minimum, impairment in reciprocal interactions with language impairment and/or restricted interests or behaviors [4]. As a result, it is a catchall diagnosis including children with a wide range of language skills, cognitive abilities, and levels of functional impairment.

Social communication and language deficits in children who have autistic spectrum disorder

Because of the increasingly broad nature of symptoms that now are included under the autism spectrum, language deficits in ASD vary dramatically across the different diagnoses and also within a single diagnostic category. Most, but not all, children who have ASD have receptive and expressive language impairments. As is the case with many developmental disorders (eg, specific language impairment), the prevalence of ASD is higher in boys than in girls. For autism, the ratio is about 3 or 4:1, but this ratio approaches about 10:1 for Asperger's disorder [1]. Unique deficits in social or pragmatic aspects of communication distinguish the communication impairments in ASD from other developmental disorders [9]. These impairments manifest differently in children of different developmental levels and across the autism spectrum. Thus, evaluations of children for ASD always must include assessments of language and social communication abilities in light of the child's cognitive level [10]. Early and appropriate diagnosis of ASD in young children requires knowledge of typical developmental milestones of language development and social communication, especially preverbal communication. Research on very young children who have ASD has focused on impairments of joint attention (the sharing of an experience, affect, or intention with another person through coordination of gaze and gesture or vocalization) as an important early sign of the social communication deficits in ASD [11]. Current guidelines and available screening tools for ASD in the first 2 years of life tap these early nonverbal communicative skills that involve joint attention deficits and apparent lack of receptive language skills [12]. The milder the early symptoms of ASD are, the more subtle the deficits in social communication may be, delaying diagnosis.

Language in toddlers and preschoolers

Typically developing infants are competent communicators well before they speak their first words. The development of joint attention and the sharing of experiences during the first year of life are critical prerequisites for more complex forms of social communication [13]. By the age of 9 to 12 months, infants develop gaze-monitoring and social-referencing skills, or the ability to observe others' focus of attention or affect by shifting gaze between people and objects [14]. This ability is seen, for example, when a baby "reads" her parent's face in a pediatrician's office to look for an indication of whether this strange adult is safe. In the same period, infants acquire understanding of gestures, single words, and phrases, initially in the context of social games or routines. They start using simple gestures or vocalizations to communicate requests or comment by reaching, pushing away, calling out, or waving. Around the first birthday, babies can respond to joint attention by following another's point to look at the object indicated, point to indicate an object, and later point so show or share an experience with another person [15,16].

Development of language comprehension and expression follow nonverbal precursors to spoken language. By the first birthday, most children say their first words and can understand many more words and some phrases. Initially meaning is linked to context, and children learn names of objects only in a single setting [17]. Between 12 and 18 months of age, there is a gradual growth in receptive and expressive vocabulary, with increasing freedom from context, and sometimes overgeneralization of words that are known (eg, any gray-haired woman is "grandma"). Around 18 months, they can "read" others' communicative intentions through eye gaze and gestures [18]. From 18 to 24 months, children have an explosive increase in vocabulary and an understanding of communicative norms such as the back-and-forth of a conversational exchange [19]. During the second year of life, in concert with increasing complexity of communication skills, toddlers have more complex play skills, advancing from constructive to functional to imaginary play, imitating actions they have seen and using them in the context of play. By the second birthday, most children have hundreds of words that are not tied to use in specific context and start putting together simple phrases or "sentences" of two or three words [20].

This predictable developmental progression goes awry in ASD. Most toddlers who have ASD have delays in acquiring language and significantly decreased vocal output [21]. Acquisition of language is slower than in other children who have language delays, often is related directly to cognitive level, but may lag behind development in other areas [22]. Children who have ASD typically use words to label, request, or protest, as a way of regulating their environment, rather than for purely social reasons, such as to comment or to initiate a social interaction [23]. Some children remain nonverbal, although as more children are identified early and receive intensive early intervention from the time of diagnosis, that number seems to be dropping [9]. It is unclear whether some of the improvement in outcome may result from diagnosis of children who have milder symptoms from the outset. Some children who have ASD and who never acquire spoken language may also have apraxia, or oral-motor impairment, impacting their ability to communicate verbally [9]. Usually, receptive language also is impaired in ASD and often seems to lag behind expressive language, although this unusual profile may reflect difficulties in testing young children's comprehension because of their lack of social responsiveness [24]. Children who have stronger language comprehension tend to have more advanced play skills and better comprehension of social interactions [25].

Babbling and other vocalizations that are present are often unusual in tone, including repetitive screeching, groaning, humming, "raspberries," or echolalia. Echolalia can be immediate or delayed, and most children who have ASD and who speak use echolalia early in language acquisition, but its frequency decreases with time. Some typically developing children also have transient immediate echolalia as a means of learning and consolidating vocabulary, and it sometimes is observed in children who are language delayed or blind [26]. Immediate echolalia can consist of the final word of another person's sentence or a complete sentence, demonstrating the characteristic pronoun reversal often seen in, although not unique to, autism (eg, a child's saying, "You want juice?" after being asked if he wants juice). Delayed echolalia can be taken from video, books, or past conversations (eg, the child's finding an adult and saying, "Are you sleepy?" to indicate he wants to nap). It is not uncommon for a child who has ASD with little or no spontaneous language to repeat commercials or large chunks or dialogue from movies. In clinical practice, parents sometimes describe "imaginary" play of their child who has autism, which consists of using toys to act out dialogue repeated verbatim from a previously watched video. Echolalic phrases may be complex but usually are uttered as a chunk, as if a single word. Although echolalia in children who have ASD seems to be a vocal stereotypy or self-stimulatory behavior, it sometimes is functional, allowing children to make requests, self-soothe, participate in a social routine or interaction, or gain time to process language [27].

Up to a quarter of children who have ASD have regression of language between the age of 12 and 18 months. In most of these children there is not a dramatic loss of language in the midst of normal language development. Usually the child uses single words inconsistently, and they gradually disappear [28]. At the same time, parents often report social withdrawal and constriction of affect or change in temperament. Regression of language and social relatedness of this sort is unique to autism and should be responded to promptly in the pediatric setting. Regression of motor or other streams of development should raise concerns of other disorders, such as childhood disintegrative disorder, neurodegenerative or metabolic disorders, or seizure disorders such as Landau-Kleffner syndrome.

Young children who have ASD demonstrate reduced use of the nonverbal communicative behaviors that precede spoken language in typically developing children. Affected children use fewer gestures, show decreased use of gaze to indicate and interpret meaning, and do not initiate or respond to bids for joint attention. Unlike other children who have language delays, children who have ASD do not compensate for their lack of speech with gestures [21]. Rather than using symbolic gestures like pointing or waving, affected children may use gestures associated with physical contact such as leading, pushing, or moving another's hand to a desired object. Problem behaviors such as aggression, self-injury, and tantrums can serve communicative functions in children on the spectrum.

Impairments in joint attention are now part of the *DSM* criteria for autism ("lack of showing, bringing, or pointing out objects of interest"). Individuals who have ASD rarely communicate for purely social reasons or enjoyment. Young children who have ASD do not show the usual precursors to joint attention, such as social referencing, sharing affect, following the gaze of another, or pointing [29]. Children who have ASD often are described by parents as being "in their own world" and do not attend to voices around them, although they usually respond to other nonvocal auditory stimuli. Typical children learn words by hearing them used in a social context, which requires joint attention. When young children not respond to social stimuli, they miss vital learning opportunities for developing language. When they do not monitor others' gaze, they may make incorrect associations between objects and words [30]. Thus impairment in joint attention may be a primary deficit that leads to delays in language.

Play in autism is atypical, usually perseverative, and lacking in imaginative themes. Several studies have found that children who have autism also have impairments in imitation [31]. Typical children learn socially by observing and imitating what they see around them, developing symbolic play that later is elaborated into imaginary play. Young children on the autistic spectrum demonstrate more solitary play including sensory exploration of toys and other objects, constructive play (eg, lining up or stacking), and trial-and-error learning of how things work. Higher levels of play in ASD correlate with expressive language level, suggesting that these children may use language skills to mediate play skills [32].

Language in school-aged children and beyond

By the time typical children enter school, they are able to speak fluently, have acquired a rich vocabulary, and use full sentences. In the early school years, children master the more complex grammatical structures of their native language; however, vocabulary continues to grow throughout the lifespan. Pragmatic and discourse skills continue to develop as children become more effective communicators, becoming more sensitive to their listener's perspective and telling more complex and well-structured narratives [33].

Many children who have ASD still have very limited language by the time they enter kindergarten, and their impairments in nonverbal communication also persist [34]. These deficits in social communication are a significant barrier to learning and may lead to increased problem behaviors. At this stage it is quite common to introduce minimally verbal children who have ASD to alternative communication systems such as manual signs or the Picture Exchange Communication System [35]. It is crucial to focus on developing language skills in young children who have ASD because the presence of speech before age 5 years is the strongest predictor for better outcomes [36].

There is considerable variability in the rate at which language progresses among verbal children who have ASD. Children with higher levels of IQ, receptive language, imitation, and joint attention skills tend to make greater gains [11]. In general, verbal children who have ASD do not have problems with articulating speech sounds [37]. They also can score quite highly on tests of vocabulary knowledge, although they may not understand or use words referring to emotions, thoughts, and other mental states [38]. Sometimes children or adults will use idiosyncratic words or phrases or made-up words (eg, "cuts and bluesers"), and their speech might be quite perseverative [39]. With respect to grammatical knowledge, there are different subgroups, with some children achieving average or above-average scores on standardized tests (about 25% of verbal children who have ASD), but the majority remains delayed [37]. Like children who have specific language impairment, children who have ASD who have impaired language have particular difficulty mastering grammatical morphology, especially for marking tense (eg, using "-ed" to construct the past tense, as in "John painted the house") and related complex syntactic structures [40].

Compared with other groups of children who have language impairment or mental retardation, the receptive language skills of children who have ASD seem to be relatively lower than their expressive skills [41]. Part of their difficulties in understanding language stem from limitations in the ability to integrate linguistic input with real-world knowledge, which may include their impaired understanding of the social world [25]. Another source of difficulty is the use of different types of cues to decipher the intended meaning of another person's message. For example, children who have ASD have core impairments integrating nonverbal cues to help interpret verbal messages, especially in everyday social interactions [42]. Thus, they may not use facial expressions, body language, or intonation to determine whether a speaker's intended message is affectionate, hostile, or teasing. Elliptical utterances, indirect requests (eg, "Can you take the garbage out?") and non-literal language (eg, lies or ironic jokes) all depend on the ability to interpret intended meaning and thus may contribute to the overall comprehension difficulties experienced by children and adults who have ASD [43].

The speech of children and adults who have ASD usually sounds odd or unusual, and this oddity is one of the immediately recognizable clinical signs of the disorder. Defining the specific abnormalities so that clinicians could make reliable judgments has been quite challenging, however, perhaps because there are many different ways in which their language sounds peculiar. These abnormalities in intonation may be even more prevalent among people who have Asperger's disorder and include flat, monotonic, or sing-song speech, nasal or high-pitched vocal tone, lack of affective quality, poor control of volume, and atypical stress patterns in words and sentences [44]. Problems with intonation are found in both expressive and receptive language: children who have ASD have difficulty distinguishing different stress patterns or interpreting emotional prosody [45].

At the heart of the language problems found in everyone who has ASD are difficulties in the area of language pragmatics, the ability to use language effectively in a variety of social contexts [9]. Children who have ASD use language in limited ways, rarely to comment, request information, acknowledge their listener, or to describe events [46]. They may fail to follow politeness rules, make irrelevant remarks, and in conversations with other people have problems taking turns and may talk either too much or too little [7]. When asked to narrate events from their lives or stories, children who have autism often include irrelevant or inappropriate content and have difficulty taking into account their listener's needs (eg, by failing to establish clear reference or by presenting events in a confused or disorganized way) [47]. These pragmatic problems seriously impede the social adaptation of both children and adults who have ASD and can lead to disruptive behavior in the classroom, on the playground, or in employment situations.

Clinical implications and recommendations

Although many parents have attributed their children's onset of symptoms to immunizations at the age of 15 months (cf. [48]), retrospective analyses of first birthday party home videotapes have shown signs of impairment of social relatedness and communication before that time [49–51]. Usually there is no period of unequivocally normal development, although abnormalities may not be noted unless regression occurs or language skills lag far behind peers, usually between 18 and 24 months [52]. Numerous studies have shown significant delays from first parental concern that "something is wrong," to referral to a specialist for evaluation, to diagnosis [53]. With improved awareness in both lay and professional communities of the early signs of autism, the interval between recognition of symptoms and diagnosis is dropping. Despite this improvement, several recent studies have shown disparities in age of diagnosis based on socioeconomic factors including ethnicity, rural residence, and income. [54] This disparity has important clinical implications, because there is ample evidence that early and intensive therapy in young children who have ASD positively impacts outcomes in language and cognition in many children [55]. Parent advocacy groups have been promoting a sense of urgency for early diagnosis of autism because of the promise of better outcomes with treatment. Routine pediatric visits are the most appropriate place for identification of early signs of ASD. It is critical for pediatric providers to be familiar with the earliest signs of impaired social communication in ASD and with screening recommendations.

A number of different studies have identified some of the earliest observable signs of ASD [56]. Not surprisingly, the findings are most robust in children who are most severely affected, who can be diagnosed earliest. The retrospective studies of parental report and home video studies mentioned previously showed decreased social interactions, less social smiling, decreased range of facial expressions, lack of response to name, decreased pointing and showing, fewer vocalizations, decreased orientation to faces, and decreased imitation [49–51]. A number of screening tools have been developed to identify ASD before 24 months. These tools include many of these early signs and have found that they discriminate between ASD and other developmental disorders, such as language or cognitive impairments [57–60]. More recently, a number of centers have initiated longitudinal studies of infants at high risk for ASD, younger siblings of children already diagnosed, who have an approximately 10% risk or higher of being on the autism spectrum. To date, initial reports from those studies have shown differences at 12 months in children later diagnosed as having ASD in the following behavior patterns: decreased receptive language; use of fewer gestures; atypical eye contact, visual tracking, and visual attention; impaired orientation to name; decreased imitation; decreased social smiling and social interest; and temperamental differences [61,62] Interestingly, siblings who were not later diagnosed as having ASD also used fewer gestures than controls [21].

Prospective research is revealing signs of ASD at the first birthday, and screening guidelines are beginning to reflect these advances. The challenge for pediatric providers lies in distinguishing children for whom language delay is a sign of the late talker from one whose language delay requires remediation. In children who require further assessment and treatment, language delay may be a symptom of developmental language disorder, global developmental delay, or ASD. Screening guidelines and tools point to ways in which these distinctions can be made in the primary care setting. The American Academy of Neurology and the Child Neurology Society published a practice parameter for screening and diagnosis of autism, including red flags requiring immediate referral for further evaluation that focus on expressive and nonverbal communication, joint attention, and regression: no babbling, or pointing, or other gestures by 12 months; no single words by 16 months; no two-word spontaneous (not echolalic) phrases at 24 months; and any loss of any language or social skills at any age [63].

The most recent guidelines for screening for developmental disorders in the pediatric setting were published by the American Academy of Pediatrics [64]. Although the algorithm is for general developmental screening, ASD figures prominently. The recommendations include routine developmental surveillance as part of every well-child visit and administration of formal screening tests during three visits in the first 3 years of life. The first formal screening is at the 9-month visit, when the provider is urged to evaluate nonverbal communication for early symptoms of autism, such as decreased eye contact, response to name, and pointing. At the 18-month visit, an autism-specific screening tool is recommended, because more general screening tools have not been found to have adequate sensitivity and specificity to identify ASD. Proposed federal legislation would mandate universal screening for autism, potentially transforming this algorithm into a standard of care.

Pediatricians are increasingly expected to recognize the subtle, early signs of ASD, before language delay is evident, and to respond quickly with appropriate referrals. Pediatricians should familiarize themselves with screening tools designed specifically to identify autism and should know how to refer parents to community resources, including specialists with expertise in ASD and early intervention programs. In addition, it is vital to have a particularly high index of suspicion in siblings of children who have ASD, especially those who have language delay, because their risk for the disorder is many times that of the general population.

Because children who have ASD face new challenges with each transition they make, first into preschool programs and then into elementary school, it is important to continue to monitor their progress to ensure that their behavioral and language needs are being addressed in their educational programs [65]. Most children who have ASD need to have their language skills assessed on a regular basis to evaluate their receptive and expressive abilities and also, importantly, their pragmatic skills. It is important to recognize that ASDs are lifelong disorders, and although significant gains in language can be expected, especially during early childhood, difficulties in effective communication that are closely tied to their core social deficits continue to require close monitoring and referrals for comprehensive evaluation and treatment.

References

[1] Volkmar F, Klin A, et al. Issues in the classification of autism and related conditions. In: Volkmar F, Paul R, Klin A, editors. Handbook of autism and pervasive developmental disorder, vol. 1. 3rd edition. New York: Wiley; 2005. p. 5–41.

[2] Klin A, McPartland J, Volkmar F, et al. Asperger syndrome. In: Volkmar F, Paul R, Klin A, editors. Handbook of autism and pervasive developmental disorder, vol. 1. 3rd edition. New York: Wiley; 2005. p. 88–125.

[3] Ozonoff S, Griffith E. Neuropsychological function and the external validity of Asperger syndrome. In: Klin A, Volkmar F, Sparrow S, editors. Asperger syndrome. New York: Guilford Press; 2000. p. 72–96.

[4] American Psychiatric Association. Diagnostic and statistical manual of mental disorders. 4th (revised) edition. Washington, DC: American Psychiatric Association; 2000.

[5] Tager-Flusberg H. Language and communicative deficits and their effects on learning and behavior. In: Prior M, editor. Asperger syndrome: behavioral and educational aspects. New York: Guilford Press; 2003. p. 85–103.

[6] Ghaziuddin M, Gerstein L. Pedantic speaking style differentiates Asperger syndrome from high-functioning autism. J Autism Dev Disord 1996;26:585–95.

[7] Landa R. Social language use in Asperger syndrome and high-functioning autism. In: Klin A, Volkmar F, Sparrow S, editors. Asperger syndrome. New York: Guilford Press; 2000. p. 125–55.

[8] Wing L. Asperger's syndrome: a clinical account. J Autism Dev Disord 1981;9:11–29.

[9] Tager-Flusberg H, Paul R, Lord CE, et al. Language and communication in autism. In: Volkmar F, Paul R, Klin A, editors. Handbook of autism and pervasive developmental disorder, vol. 1. 3rd edition. New York: Wiley; 2005. p. 335–64.

[10] Paul R, et al. Assessing communication in autism spectrum disorders. In: Volkmar F, Paul R, Klin A, editors. Handbook of autism and pervasive developmental disorder, vol. 2. 3rd edition. New York: Wiley; 2005. p. 799–816.

[11] Sigman M, Ruskin E. Continuity and change in the social competence of children with autism, Down syndrome and developmental delays. Monographs of the Society for Research in Child Development 1999;64(Serial No. 256).

[12] Zwaigenbaum L, Stone W. Early screening for autism spectrum disorders in clinical practice settings. In: Charman T, Stone W, editors. Social and communication development in autism spectrum disorders: early identification, diagnosis, and intervention. New York: Guilford Press; 2006. p. 88–113.

[13] Carpenter M, Nagell K, Tomasello M. Social cognition, joint attention, and communicative competence from 9 to 15 months of age. Monographs of the Society for Research in Child Development 1998'63(Serial No. 255).

[14] Hertenstein M, Campos J. The retention effects of an adult's emotional displays on infant behavior. Child Dev 2004;75:595–613.

[15] Bates E. Language in context. New York: Academic Press; 1976.

[16] Bruner J. The social context of language acquisition. Lang Commun 1981;1:155–78.

[17] Tomasello M, Kruger AC. Joint attention on actions: acquiring verbs in ostensive and non-ostensive contests. J Child Lang 1992;19:311–33.

[18] Baldwin DA. Infants' contribution to the achievement of joint reference. Child Dev 1991;62: 875–90.

[19] Fenson L, Dale P, Reznick J, et-al. Variability in early communicative development. Monographs of the Society for Research in Child Development 1994;59 (Serial No. 242).

[20] Brown R. A first language. Cambridge (UK): Harvard University Press; 1973.

[21] Mitchell S, Brian J, Zwaigenbaum L, et al. Early language and communication development of infants later diagnosed with autism spectrum disorder. J Dev Behav Pediatr 2006;27: S69–78.

[22] Lord C, Pickles A. The relationship between expressive language level and nonverbal social communication in autism. J Am Acad Child Adolesc Psychiatry 1996;35:1542–50.

[23] Wetherby A. Ontogeny of communication functions in autism. J Autism Dev Disord 1986; 16:295–316.

[24] Rutter M, Mawhood L, Howlin P. Language delay and social development. In: Fletcher P, Hall D, editors. Specific speech and language disorders in children: correlates, characteristics and outcomes. London: Whurr Publishers; 1992. p. 63–78.

[25] Lord C. Autism and the comprehension of language. In: Schopler E, Mesibov G, editors. Communication problems in autism. New York: Plenum; 1985. p. 257–81.

[26] Hobson RP. Why connect? On the relation between autism and blindness. In: Pring L, editor. Autism and blindness: research and reflections. London: Whurr Publishers Ltd; 2005. p. 10–25.

[27] Prizant BM. Echolalia in autism: assessment and intervention. Semin Speech Lang 1983;4: 63–77.

[28] Luyster R, Richler J, Risi S, et al. Early regression in social communication in autistic spectrum disorders. Dev Neuropsychol 2005;27:311–36.

[29] Lord C, Richler J. Early diagnosis of children with autism spectrum disorders. In: Charman T, Stone W, editors. Social and communication development in autism spectrum disorders: early identification, diagnosis, and intervention. New York: Guilford Press; 2006. p. 35–59.

[30] Baron-Cohen S, Baldwin DA, Crowson M. Do children with autism use the speaker's direction of gaze strategy to crack to code of language? Child Dev 1997;68:48–57.

[31] Rogers S, Stackhouse T, Hepburn S, et al. Imitation performance in toddlers with autism and those with other developmental disorders. J Child Psychol Psychiatry 2003;44:763–81.

[32] Rogers S, Cook I, Meryl D, et al. Imitation and play in autism. In: Volkmar F, Paul R, Klin A, editors. Handbook of autism and pervasive developmental disorder, vol. 1. 3rd edition. New York: Wiley; 2005. p. 382–405.

[33] Ely R. Language and literacy in the school years. In: Gleason JB, editor. The development of language. 6th edition. Boston: Allyn & Bacon; 2005. p. 396–443.

[34] Loveland K, Landry S. Joint attention and communication in autism and language delay. J Autism Dev Disord 1986;16:335–49.

[35] Bondy A, Frost L. The picture exchange communication system. Semin Speech Lang 1998; 19:373–89.

[36] Rutter M. Autistic children: infancy to adulthood. Semin Psychiatry 1970;2:435–50.

[37] Kjelgaard M, Tager-Flusberg H. An investigation of language impairment in autism: implications for genetic subgroups. Lang Cogn Process 2001;16:287–308.

[38] Hobson RP, Lee A. Emotion-related and abstract concepts in autistic people: evidence from the British Picture Vocabulary Scale. J Autism Dev Disord 1989;19:601–23.

[39] Volden J, Lord C. Neologisms and idiosyncratic language in autistic speakers. J Autism Dev Disord 1991;21:109–30.

[40] Roberts J, Rice M, Tager-Flusberg H. Tense marking in children with autism. Appl Psycholinguist 2004;25:429–48.

[41] Tager-Flusberg H. On the nature of linguistic functioning in early infantile autism. J Autism Dev Disord 1981;11:45–56.

[42] Loveland KA. Social affordances and interaction: II. Autism and the affordances of the human environment. Ecological Psychology 1991;3:99–119.

[43] Paul R, Cohen DJ. Comprehension of indirect requests in adults with mental retardation and pervasive developmental disorders. J Speech Hear Res 1985;28:475–9.

[44] Shriberg L, Paul R, McSweeney J, et al. Speech and prosody characteristics of adolescents and adults with high-functioning autism and Asperger syndrome. J Speech Lang Hear Res 2001;44:1097–115.

[45] Koning C, Magill-Evans J. Social and language skills in adolescent boys with Asperger syndrome. Autism 2001;5:23–36.

[46] Wetherby AM, Prutting CA. Profiles of communicative and cognitive-social abilities in autistic children. J Speech Hear Res 1984;27:364–77.

[47] Loveland KA, McEvoy RE, Tunali B, et al. Narrative story telling in autism and Down syndrome. British Journal of Developmental Psychology 1990;8:9–23.

[48] Fombonne E, Zakarian R, Bennett A, et al. Pervasive developmental disorders in Montreal, Quebec, Canada: prevalence and links with immunizations. Pediatrics 2006;118:e139–50.

[49] Adrien J, Lenoir P, Martineau J, et al. Blind ratings of early symptoms of autism based upon family home movies. J Am Acad Child Adolesc Psychiatry 1993;32:617–26.

[50] Baranek G. Autism during infancy: a retrospective video analysis of sensory-motor and social behaviors at 9–12 months of age. J Autism Dev Disord 1999;29:213–24.

[51] Osterling J, Dawson G, Munson J. Early recognition of 1-year-old infants with autism spectrum disorder versus mental retardation. Development and Psychopathology 2002;14: 239–51.

[52] Lord C, Shulman C, DiLavore P. Regression and word loss in autistic spectrum disorders. J Child Psychol Psychiatry 2004;45:936–55.

[53] Charman T, Baron-Cohen S. Screening for autism spectrum disorders in populations: progress, challenges, and questions for future research and practice. In: Charman T, Stone W, editors. Social and communication development in autism spectrum disorders: early identification, diagnosis, and intervention. New York: Guilford Press; 2006. p. 63–87.

[54] Mandell D, Novak M, Zubritsky C. Factors associated with age of diagnosis among children with autism spectrum disorders. Pediatrics 2005;116:1480–6.

[55] NRC. Educating children with autism. Washington, DC: National Academy Press; 2001.

[56] Charman T, Baird G. Practitioner review: diagnosis of autism spectrum disorder in 2- and 3-year-old children. J Child Psychol Psychiatry 2002;43:289–305.

[57] Robins D, Fein D, Barton M, et al. The modified checklist for autism in toddlers: an initial study investigating the early detection of autism and pervasive developmental disorders. J Autism Dev Disord 2001;31:131–44.

[58] Siegel B. The pervasive developmental disorders screening Test-II (PDDST-II). San Antonio (TX): Psychological Corporation; 2004.

[59] Stone W, Coonrod E, Turner L, et al. Psychometric properties of the STAT for early autism screening. J Autism Dev Disord 2004;34:691–701.

[60] Wetherby A, Woods J, Allen L, et al. Early indicators of autism spectrum disorders in the second year of life. J Autism Dev Disord 2004;34:473–93.

[61] Landa R, Garrett-Mayer E. Development in infants with autism spectrum disorders: a prospective study. J Child Psychol Psychiatry 2006;47:629–38.

[62] Zwaigenbaum L, Bryson S, Rogers T, et al. Behavioral markers of autism in the first year of life. International Journal of Developmental Neurosciences 2005;23:143–52.

[63] Filipek P, Accardo P, Ashwal S, et al. Practice parameter: screening and diagnosis of autism. Report of the Quality Standards Subcommittee of the American Academy of Neurology and the Child Neurology Society. Neurology 2000;55:468–79.

[64] Council on Children with Disabilities, Section on Developmental Behavioral Pediatrics, Bright Futures Steering Committee, Medical Home Initiatives for Children With Special

Needs Project Advisory Committee. Identifying infants and young children with developmental disorders in the medical home: an algorithm for developmental surveillance and
screening. Pediatrics 2006;118:405–20.

[65] Marans W, Rubin E, Laurent A, et al. Addressing social communication skills in individuals
with high-functionign autism and Asperger syndrome: critical priorities in educational programming. In: Volkmar F, Paul R, Klin A, editors. Handbook of autism and pervasive
developmental disorder, vol. 2. 3rd edition. New York: Wiley; 2005. p. 977–1002.

ELSEVIER
SAUNDERS

PEDIATRIC CLINICS
OF NORTH AMERICA

Pediatr Clin N Am 54 (2007) 483–506

Social Communication Impairments: Pragmatics

Robert L. Russell, PhD[a,b,*]

[a]Medical College of Wisconsin, 8701 Watertown Plank Road, PO Box 26509,
Milwaukee, WI 53226–0509, USA
[b]Child Development Center, MEB, Children's Hospital of Wisconsin,
9000 W. Wisconsin Avenue, Milwaukee, WI 53226–0509, USA

When one hears or reads a sentence, it is often easy to determine if it is syntactically correct, if it makes sense or is coherent semantically, and if the words are pronounced or pronounceable in a phonetically acceptable way. Further, it is not often difficult to determine if a spoken sentence seems acceptable or correct in terms of its prosody, as when a statement is said as a question with a rising intonation pattern (eg, That was an owl?) or when words in the sentence are said too fast or slow, or too loud or soft. In many cases, the determination of the syntactic well-formedness of a sentence, its semantic interpretation, and the correctness of the pronunciation and prosody can be made without use of extrasentential information (eg, other utterances that surround the target utterance, the context in which it occurred, the speaker's and listener's intentions). Informally, native knowledge of language is used to make these judgments of correctness, even if it is difficult to specify exactly what aspect of a sentence sounds correct or incorrect or what rule has been correctly followed or violated. Usually, these judgments are made on a holistic basis: either the sentence sounds acceptable and well-formed or it does not. Formally, such native knowledge is also used in assessing a child's expressive and receptive language abilities, but it is augmented and considered in combination with standardized language and speech tests and measurements.

The central topic of this article, however, concerns how speaker's use their language and gestures to meet their and others' interactional goals in the contexts that comprise their everyday life. This topic is often described

* Medical College of Wisconsin, 8701 Watertown Plank Road, PO Box 26509, Milwaukee, WI 53226–0509.
E-mail address: rrussell@mcw.edu

0031-3955/07/$ - see front matter © 2007 Published by Elsevier Inc.
doi:10.1016/j.pcl.2007.02.016

with various terms, such as social communication competence, sociolinguistic competence, ethnography of communication, or pragmatics [1–3]. The focus here is on the development of, and impairments in, pragmatics [1,4–7]. From the perspective of pragmatics, judgments about syntax, semantics, and even aspects of phonetics and prosody depend importantly on knowledge about the specific occasion in which the words were uttered or written, about the intentions of the speaker or writer in producing the utterance, and about the discourses or genres in which they are embedded. When interested in social communication by language or gesture, one can ask about the form, the meaning, the phonetic pronunciation, and the prosody of a particular isolated sentence, but this rather misses the point. In social communication, one is less interested in structural aspects of words and sentences and more interested in the contextual meanings they convey and how they function appropriately or inappropriately effectively to meet interpersonal and behavioral goals. One is interested in meanings that are intended by speakers as they converse and gesture in specific historical and communication circumstances. In trying to understand pragmatics, the goal is "to explain how the gap between sentence meaning and speaker's meaning is bridged" [8].

When trying to decipher speaker meaning, one is required to consider aspects of development, biography, and subculture, in addition to linguistics. These often extrasentential considerations provide the basis for deciphering the meaning and appropriateness of the gestures, discourses, and stories that individuals create to express themselves (eg, I feel wonderful today); carry out social actions (eg, promises, bets, avowals); and establish a consensus about what is held to be true. Conversely, speakers who have developed communicative competence must have knowledge about rather complex extrasentential and extralinguistic states of affairs (eg, status of interlocutors, rules of politeness and address, cultural norms) to select from a repertoire of linguistic forms just the right ones that advance their interpersonal and behavioral needs while preserving a sense of social order for all those involved in the communication event.

Another way to highlight what is of interest when attempting to assess social communication competence, as opposed to linguistic competence, is to remember that the communicative use of language and gesture in context is a form of interpersonal action. People do things with words [9,10]. Social communication is symbolic action, typically sequenced in relation to others' symbolic actions, which together comprise important aspects of the communication event [11,12]. This is why it is essential to ask a set of questions that seem inappropriate or superfluous if one's interest is solely in making judgments about the grammaticality, semantics, and phonology of sentences. Consider the following questions. What is the speaker doing in saying "X"? Is what the speaker doing in saying "X" appropriate for the situation, the listener, and even for himself or herself? Does the listener recognize what the speaker is doing in saying "X," and is the listener impacted or affected in ways that the speaker does and does not intend? Are the gestures and language that the speaker uses in saying and doing "X" effective, normative, legitimate, and sincere? Is the speaker able to synchronize and adjust their communications to characteristics of those involved in the communication event; that is, do they seem in or out of rhythm with the natural flow of discourse and do they seem attuned to listener's cognitive level, interests, and concerns? Is the manner in which the speaker converses polite and deferent, or is the manner quarrelsome and belligerent? Is the speaker telling a coherent story, or is it truncated or sequenced in unexpected or even incomprehensible ways? Obviously, these and other related questions are quite different from those that are asked to determine if a child can form complex sentences, has the expected rate of vocabulary growth, understands verb tense and subject-verb agreement, can generate synonyms and rhymes, as is our interest when assessing expressive and receptive linguistic competence.

For example, consider the simple sentence "It's too cold here for itty-bitty bunny." The simple words that comprise this sentence are easily recognized and interpretable; they are in most children's aged 3 to 4 vocabulary. The words occur in the correct order and with the proper subject-verb agreement; that is, one recognizes the string of words as grammatical. Additionally, if the words were said out loud, one would recognize the string of sounds that had been made as representing just the right words. One can use native knowledge as a speaker of English to conclude that the sentence in all of its linguistic aspects is acceptable. One has no way to pin down what a real speaker in real time meant to do or even what he or she meant, however, by uttering just these words to a specific listener in a specific context. For example, "It" could have been used to refer to a particular thing that the speaker deems to be too cold when considered from the bunny's point of view rather than to a general atmospheric state. Further, one has no way to pin down what the speaker meant to do (or even what he or she meant) without having contextual information about comparative locales, which is necessary to understand "here." "Here" could refer to a room, but it could also refer to a playhouse or a cage in a room. With rising intonation, the speaker could have used the words to express a certain degree of incredulity in reaction to a listener's shivering gestures. Similarly, with added stress on "cold" in an exclamation, the speaker could be indirectly asking someone to close an opened window or door, especially if he or she also trained his or her gaze in their direction. Finally, if standing in front of a particularly heartless board of examiners, a condescending speaker could have meant something entirely different by the exclamation, when uttering these words to an obviously nervous fellow examinee. In this last metaphoric or figurative use of the sentence, there is no way one could arrive at the speaker's meaning, glossed as something like "These examiners' formality, exactitude, and persistence creates an uncomfortable situation for innocents like you as compared with more resilient types like me," from the semantics of the isolated sentence "It's too cold here for itty-bitty bunny."

It is important to also note, however, that the use of the noun "bunny" and the adjective "itty-bitty," instead of the more formal "rabbit" and "tiny," suggests who is speaking or to whom is being spoken. This constraint on plausible speakers, apparently associated with the two specific lexical items (itty-bitty, bunny), marks the speaker's or listener's identity as a child or someone in a childlike state, at least in the literal use of the utterance. If this is true, one can see that at least some features of the context (eg, characteristics of the speaker or listener, such as age) are even built into the broader or connoted meaning of lexical items, and this seems also to be true for aspects of syntax and semantics. Without context, for example, there is no way to pinpoint to whom pronouns refer (Can you hand the stethoscope to her?), and their meaning must remain ambiguous or indeterminate until sufficient context is provided. Importantly, one's native knowledge of language use can be and is used to assess the appropriateness of social communications in context. Again, such judgments are typically made on a holistic basis: either the communication seemed or did not seem appropriate. Such native knowledge, in conjunction with information gathered by formal testing procedures and controlled observation, can be used to identify children who have difficulties with social communication in and across the contexts that make up their daily lives.

Pragmatics, the study of the use of language and gesture in context, has not been defined in a way that has won universal acceptance among experts [1,5,7,13]. There are several important aspects of pragmatics that are obvious and noncontroversial. For example, in the working definition given previously, there is at least general agreement about certain aspects of context, language, gesture, and use. Context is of paramount importance in pragmatics. Any given communication is embedded within multiple contexts: autobiographic, biographic, developmental, interpersonal, situational, cultural, and language-gestural contexts. These contexts can be present to various degrees to the interlocutors (as when they meet in the context of a basketball game, or social studies class, or karate competition), but are more commonly in the background or presumed (as when one good friend says to another on Monday morning in homeroom: "You must be as devastated as I am" meaning "Knowing how we both feel about our Packers, I presume you too watched them lose yesterday and you, like me, feel devastated"). Note how biographic, interpersonal, and cultural knowledge, most of which is presumed rather than articulated, must be brought to bear to understand even this brief utterance, never mind the knowledge of English necessary to form the sentence. In pragmatics there is an interest in the structural features of language, but this concern is outweighed by a focus on language use, or language use as symbolic action. As a consequence, the forms of language use that are of interest no longer center on sentences (as in linguistics proper) but rather include utterances, exchanges, lectures, stories, conversations and their accompanying gestures, all of which are variously used by speakers to accomplish their goals. Evaluating an individual's pragmatic competence requires an assessment not only of the speaker's communicative repertoire (eg, the size of their vocabulary, the average length of utterance, the types of speech acts that they can make, whether they can use and understand both simple and complex sentences), but whether or not the speaker's language use is typically appropriate, legitimate, normative, successful, and sincere given the speaker's developmental level and context of interaction. Three clinical examples illustrate some of these points:

1. Ritual greeting A. A 7-year-old boy is seated in the clinic waiting room with his "mother." The clinician approaches. The clinician introduces himself: "Hello. I am Dr. Wells." Dr. Well's hand is extended toward the adult, who stands and shakes it. Dr. Wells turns to the 7 year old, who stands up and partially extends his hand toward Dr. Well's, who finds it rather limp and without a grip. "Good afternoon, Dr. Wells. I am Timothy William Smith. I believe your appointment is with me. This is my stepmother." There is only shifting eye contact between Timothy and Dr. Wells. Timothy, however, continues to talk. "We used our GPS to locate the clinic. It is 23.7 miles due East from our home. We traveled on four local streets, two state highways, and one interstate that were built when General Eisenhower was the President. How did you get here?"

2. Ritual greeting B. A 7-year-old girl is seated in the clinic waiting room with her mother. The clinician approaches. The clinician introduces himself: "Hello. I am Dr. Wells." Dr. Well's hand is extended toward the mother who stands and shakes it, introducing herself as Mrs. Smith. She turns toward her daughter, playing with a rag doll, and says: "Molly, say hello to Dr. Wells." A moment passes without any behavior. The mother repeats her request with more urgency. Molly stands up and holds her doll out to Dr. Wells. After commenting on what a nice doll Molly has, Dr. Wells suggests that they all go back to the conference room. Before Dr. Wells takes a step, Molly takes his hand, and beginning to walk, says, "Tammy. Yours," holding the doll up again for Dr. Wells to take.

3. Ritual greeting C. A 7-year-old boy is seated in the clinic waiting room with his mother. The clinician approaches. The clinician introduces himself: "Hello. I am Dr. Wells." Dr. Well's hand is extended toward the mother who stands and shakes it, introducing herself as Mrs. Smith. Mrs. Smith turns to her son and says: "Johnny, say hello to Dr. Wells." Johnny says: "Hello," with a raspy voice, but does not look up from his Gameboy when Dr. Wells says hello in response. Dr. Wells begins to suggest that they go back to the conference room but is interrupted when Johnny jumps up and quite excitedly and loudly exclaims: "I won. I won. Mom, I won." Without hesitating he next turns to Dr. Wells and waves his finger at him: "You're not going to give me a shot, are you?"

Although it would be premature to solidify a diagnostic impression on the basis of the children's participation in the ritual greeting, it is clear a normative set of pragmatic expectations is frustrated in each of the scenarios. In the first scenario, Timothy's communications seem overly formal and at the same time convey overly detailed and irrelevant information relative to the task at hand (ie, exchanging a first greeting or introduction). Further, his request for the details of Dr. Wells' route to the clinic seems somewhat intrusive, just as his edification that the person with him is his stepmother and that the appointment is with him, not her, seems somewhat insensitive or overly assertive. It should also be noted that in addition to his bid to take control of the topic, the amount and content of his talk seems to violate an expectation of the rapidity and synchrony with which ritual greetings progress. Finally, it is also inferred from his communication that this is a 7 year old with above average language skills and intelligence quotient (IQ), and that he is likely to be at risk for social isolation or ostracism if these types of pragmatic violations occur in the social contexts shared with his age peers.

The departures from conversational expectations are equally striking in Molly's case. Just as Timothy's formality and assertiveness seem both inappropriate and pseudomature developmentally for a 7 year old, Molly's paucity of verbal communication, lack of syntactic structure to her utterances, gift-giving gesturing, and over-friendliness expressed through handholding, seem developmentally immature and inappropriate for a 7 year old. She never quite completes an introduction as would be expected from a verbal exchange between a 7 year old and an adult, nor does she actually comply with her mother's two requests: "Molly, say hello to Dr. Wells." It seems that two requests were issued by Molly's mother because Molly did not respond to the first request in the expected turn-taking time frame. Because the lexical items "hello" and "goodbye" (or their diminutives) and their use in greetings and farewells are usually mastered before possessive pronouns (eg, yours), it is not unreasonable to infer that Molly at least had the lexical item "hello" in her vocabulary even though she does not actually offer a verbal greeting in an expected fashion. Moreover, the mother's request to say hello implies or implicates that Molly can in fact say hello. Finally, just as Timothy's pragmatic performance in the ritual greeting creates an impression of a child with advanced language competencies and above average IQ, Molly's pragmatic performance creates an impression of a child with limited language competencies and below average IQ.

Johnny too does not seem to complete the ritual greeting according to expectations. Several pragmatic lapses are easily noted: failure to make eye contact when issuing a greeting, interruption of an adult speaker, failure to moderate his speech volume, and failure to shift activity frames from private involvement in a game to a publicly framed greeting and adult-initiated communicative interaction. In addition, with the exception of his uttering an obligatory "hello," Johnny ignores the initiated adult conversational framing and attempts to seize conversational topic control, first with his exclamation focusing attention on his gaming prowess and second with his barely mitigated directive or threat (eg, directive plus question tag) concerning the doctor's possible intention of giving him a shot. The rapidity with which he switches topics without securing topic uptake from the adults also seems conversationally problematic in that little reciprocity is evidenced. Of note too is that Johnny's nonverbal gesturing varies from failure to make eye contact to waving his finger at Dr. Wells, the latter more often accompanying a threat than a bona fide question. Neither type of gesture (or absence thereof) seems appropriate. Although Johnny's language seems intact, his raspy voice and lack of volume control suggest a possible history of voice abuse. Unlike Molly and Timothy, Johnny's participation in the ritual greeting reveals few language-based or discourse-based clues that suggest a below or above normal IQ.

These three examples also reveal that diagnostic impressions can begin to be formed based on the quality of the children's pragmatic participation in even such a simple, well-scripted ritual as a greeting. In Timothy's case, ruling out a pervasive developmental disorder, such as Asperger's syndrome, is diagnostically reasonable. In contrast, in Molly's case, ruling out mental retardation, an expressive-receptive language disorder, and other neurodevelopmental disorders seems reasonable, if Down syndrome is not also at issue. Finally, in Johnny's case, ruling out attention deficit disorder with hyperactivity (ADHD) or oppositional defiant disorder (ODD) is reasonable. For each case, the relevant diagnostic and evaluation pathways need to be considered with other information in the case history and in the context of the presenting problem. Pragmatic impairments in social communication can provide a wealth of useful information, including diagnostic clues, if closely observed. This is not surprising given the high comorbidity of pragmatic language disorders and impairments with developmental, internalizing, and externalizing disorders (see later).

Assessing pragmatic competence: types, dimensions, milestones

The formal assessment of children's pragmatic language skill has lagged behind the assessment of children's structural language competence [6,14–16]. In the past decade, however, increased attention has been devoted to devising formal tests and behavioral checklists that can provide an estimate of the development of a child's pragmatic skills [17–29]. A sense of what types of skills are typically assessed and their relative prominence or salience has been garnered by reviewing a sample of 24 such tests and checklists, and coding the domain that seems the primary target for each test item or checklist question [30]. In addition, the relative complexity of each pragmatic skill can be grouped in terms of three broad levels of pragmatic development.

For example, Fig. 1 combines four types of information (ie, type of skill domain, relative salience or prominence of the domain in the reviewed instrument set, relative complexity and approximate relative age of the emergence of the skill domain, and progressive development within each domain). As can be seen, there are 16 domains whose relative salience is represented by the size of the slice it occupies (each slice represents the proportion of all questions or tasks of the target domain divided by all of the questions and tasks in the instruments that were reviewed). In addition, there are three color-demarcated stages of pragmatic development, which indicate in clockwise fashion the approximate relative age of the domain's emergence: precursors-enablers-protoforms, basic exchanges-rounds, and extended literal and nonliteral discourse, which cover approximately the first 4 to 5 years of development. Development within each domain and approximation to the ideal competence is represented by the increasingly lighter shade of each of the three hues from the circle's circumference to its center. It should also be noted that the progressively lighter shade of each hue also illustrates a fundamental principle: as development occurs there is a progression from a state of relative undifferentiatedness to a state of relative differentiation and integration. From a state of relative undifferentiated and primitive pragmatic skills at birth, differentiated skills develop with normal maturational and socialization processes, but as each skill undergoes further development, they are systematically integrated and organized in attaining pragmatic communicative competence.

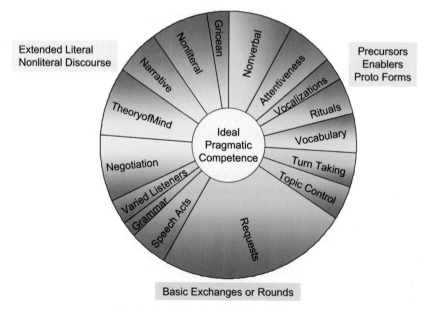

Fig. 1. Domains of pragmatic competence.

An example clarifies the illustration. In the first couple months of life, an infant trains their attention on the expressive features of the human face, the mouth and eye areas in particular. This disposition is facilitated by the exaggerated facial "gesturing" that caregivers display in the infants field of visual acuity. Moreover, the infant begins to differentially attend to vocal sounds as opposed to other environmental sounds and soon attempts to orient to the direction from which the sounds of a human voice seem to have been made. Such attention to the human voice is also facilitated by the use of the baby-talk register, with its wide pitch fluctuations, frequent repetitions, simplified syntax, and so forth. Later, infants seem to attend to particular consonants and vowels that have figured in caretaker speech and practice imitating them, sometimes in play with a caregiver and sometimes independently. It is not long before infants seem to attend to and differentiate between prosodic features of happy versus alarming communications and between word-like and non–word-like vocalizations. At the same time, infants seem to make "proto-demands" of the care-giver's attention, first as crying or whining, but later with gestures and then words, as the caregiver takes leave of the interaction or attends to something else other than the infant. Shortly thereafter, the infant-toddler's trajectory of attention development moves outward to establish a shared environment (joint attention) and inward to focus on the goal-directiveness and intentionality expressed in her and others' language use. As development continues, discourse attention is able to be trained beyond the present and bring into focus symbolic representations of events, people, and things from the past and future. Even as these basic developments in discourse attention mature, however, they seem to coalesce and involve other pragmatic domains. For example, as attention shifts from a focus on human sounds to human intentions conveyed through speech, a shift also occurs in the infant's theory of mind abilities. Likewise, as the infant's attention can span past, present, and future, a shift occurs in the form of the language they use, not just in terms of tense markings but in terms of the ability to produce and understand simple narratives. As each individual skill develops toward the ideal, it becomes more and more integrated with the other differentiated skills. For example, to differentiate a lie from a joke or even some forms of sarcasm, a listener must be able to attend to both the surface meaning of a string of words and to the speaker's beliefs about the listener's beliefs relative to some shared state of affairs relevant to the "lie" or "joke." Here attention must be able to shift effortlessly not just from spoken words to speaker intentions, but also across speaker and listener subjective biographies.

Such qualitative and quantitative developments emerge even in an area as seemingly straightforward as vocabulary development. Charting the growth in a child's vocabulary size, a relatively simple task, can provide very useful information about their language development, fluency, and beginning literacy skills. Charting increases in vocabulary size, however, is insufficient to detail the types of experiences and worlds that certain classes of words, when learned, make available and enhance. The learning of cognitive verbs (eg, think, belief, guess) and emotion words (such verbs as agonized, worried, felt; such nouns as shame, remorse, guilt, awe) helps to articulate one's inner experiences and allows them to be expressed rather than acted out. Such word learning goes hand-in-hand with and augments the development of theories of mind. Similar developments can be illustrated with the learning of the class of words called "conjunctions." Experiences and events can be verbally concatenated with the addition of "and" to a child's vocabulary; consequently, chronicles of the child's experience can be communicated. Later, with the learning of causal connectives (eg, because) and conditional connectives (if, then), relationships between events can be articulated at a much higher more complicated level. Such developments enable children to tell narratives of a form approximating that of adults. Definitions and examples of the 16 pragmatic domains featured in Fig. 1 can be found in Table 1.

Table 2 includes a sample of pragmatic and communication milestones that are roughly grouped by age of emergence or acquisition to provide an idea of normal pragmatic development [31–35]. Many of the tabled behaviors can be described in terms of the pragmatic domains included in Fig. 1 and Table 1. For example, many of the pragmatic communications that occur in the first months of life are performed nonverbally through gestures, vocalizations, and facial expressions. By 9 months of life, these forms of nonverbal communicating are well on their way to being absorbed, and thereby transformed, in the reciprocal and normative turn-taking structures associated with mature discourse and conversations. Typically, a pediatrician does not have the time or training to assess a child's pragmatic communicative competence in detail during a typical 15- to 20-minute wellness visit. Interview of the parent and observation of the child's language use, however, can provide some of the information necessary to describe the child's pragmatic skill development. Such information, along with a qualitative assessment of child's age-appropriate acquisition of the milestones, can provide a reasonable indication if more formal pragmatic language assessment is required.

The development of each of the individual pragmatic domains also entails integration and coalescence with the other pragmatic domains if the ideal of pragmatic competence is to be approximated. Such approximation can and does proceed well after grade school and through the adolescent years. In addition to the emergence, differentiation, and integration of the various pragmatic domains over the child and adolescent years, an individual's use of them in discourse can and should be described in terms of a characteristic or typical manner of interpersonal engagement.

Fig. 2 provides a sketch of one way to organize and think about an individual's characteristic manner of engaging others with their pragmatic language skills. As can be seen, the characteristic manners of pragmatic engagement are organized in terms of two axes, one that can be described

Table 1
Pragmatic modes of engagement

Precursors and enablers	Illustrative descriptions	Positive and negative examples
Nonverbal	Probes an individual's ability to attend to and understand nonverbal behavior as communicative.	Maintains eye contact, appropriate body position during conversations.
Attentiveness	Probes an individual's ability to attend to the communication partner's experience or their communications, or engage in empathic listening.	With familiar adults, seems inattentive, distant, or preoccupied.
Vocalizations	Probes an individual's ability to make speech sounds, articulate appropriately, or to use prosody	Can vary their tone of voice.
Rituals	Probes an individual's ability to participate in communicative games, use typical greetings and farewells, terms of address, and ritualistic politeness formulas (eg, please and thank you).	Makes and responds to greetings to and from others.
Vocabulary	Probes an individual's ability to use vocabulary appropriately or to evidence appropriate understanding and use of a certain number or class of words.	Uses words to express their feelings.
Comprehensibility	Probes an individual's ability to engage in understandable communicative discourse.	It is hard to make sense of what he or she is saying even though the words are clearly spoken.
Basic exchanges and rounds		
Turn taking	Probes an individual's ability to take turns in a communicative exchange, and to assume conversational roles of speaker and listener in an appropriate manner.	Observes turn-taking rules in the classroom or in social interactions.
Topic control	Probes an individual's ability to initiate, maintain, or change topics	Maintains topics using appropriate strategies.
Requests	Probes an individual's ability to formulate requests, questions of various form, and answers	Asks for and responds to requests for clarification during conversations.
Speech acts	Probes an individual's ability to select among and use a variety of speech acts	Apologizes and accepts apologies appropriately.

(*continued on next page*)

Table 1 (*continued*)

Precursors and enablers	Illustrative descriptions	Positive and negative examples
Grammar	Probes an individual's ability to formulate grammatical sentences, use proper tenses, or have subject and verbs agree	Leaves off past tense ("ed" endings on words).
Varied listeners	Probes an individual's ability to communicate with a variety of communication partners in a variety of circumstances.	Adjust or modifies language based on the communication situation.
Extended literal and nonliteral discourse		
Negotiation	Probes an individual's ability to negotiate in conversation and provide directions, instructions, or recipes.	Can disagree appropriately and offer compromises.
Theory of mind	Probes an individual's ability to use internal state cognitive or emotional language; cognitive or emotional perspective taking; or attributions of intentions, desires, and so forth.	Offers and responds to expressions of affection or belief appropriately.
Narrative	Probes an individual's ability to use narratives, stories, scripts, or descriptions in their communicative discourse.	Gets the sequence of events muddled up when trying to tell a story.
Nonliteral	Probes an individual's ability to use indirect or nonliteral expressions, or to use and understand presupposed knowledge in communication	Understands implied group and school rules.
Gricean	Probes an individual's ability to abide the core set of Gricean maxims of quantity (be informative but not more than necessary), quality (do not say what you know is false or what you lack evidence for), relation (be relevant), and manner (avoid obscurity and ambiguity, be brief and orderly), each in accord with the principle of co-operativeness (make your conversational contribution fitting to the accepted purpose or direction of current talk).	Tells people things they already know.

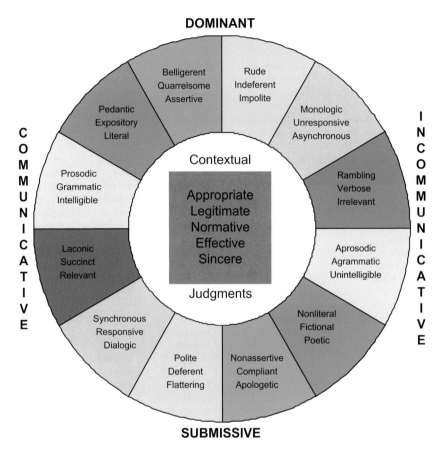

Fig. 2. Pragmatic dimensions of utterances.

as the dominant-submissive axis and one that can be described as the communicative-incommunicative axis. Complimentary manners of pragmatic engagement share the same hue and are located directly across the circle from each other. For example, literal, expository, pedantic manners of engagement are complimentary to and across the circle from nonliteral, fictional, poetic manners of engagement. It should also be evident that each of the 12 moments of the circle contains three prototypical manners of engagement that differ from each other by their degree of extremity. For example, "belligerent" is a more extreme, dominating form of discourse engagement than "quarrelsome," which is a more extreme, dominating form of discourse engagement than "assertive."

It should be noted that neither the 12 moments nor their prototypes are mutually exclusive; that is, an individual's characteristic manner of engagement may be best described by combining different moments and

Table 2
Developmental milestones relevant to pragmatic communication

Month 1	Months 2–4	Month 6	Months 9–12	Months 12–18	Months 18–24
Quiets in response to sound	Coos Turns at cooing	Responds to name Recognizes familiar faces/ people Babbles/ phonological play/vocalizes with intonation	Bye-bye Points "Mama" Coughs/laughs to attract attention Shakes head "no"	Follows verbal commands First words Jargon Points to body parts, objects	Comprehends simple sentences Word learning is fast – vocabulary 150–300
Preference for human voice	Smiles in response to smiles				
Preference/ interest in human face: looks at people	Fixes gaze on face Looks for source of voice	Responds to human voice intention without visual cues	Affectionate to familiars Pats, pulls, tugs on humans Responds to pointing	Word learning – slow Practices inflection Aware of social value of speech	Two word phrases, noun + verb, MLU 1.2 Simple object names
Cries – different cries	Expresses frustration, surprise	Differentiates between tones in angry and friendly communications	Participates in peek a boo and vocal play	Says "no," pushes objects away	Uses: in, or, under Verbal turn- taking –
Follows moving person with eyes		Initiates vocalization to person Enjoys play Cries when parent leaves	Uses proto- declaratives (statements) Uses proto- imperatives (requests)	Shows objects to adults Solicits attention vocally and verbally	a few turns on a single topic Rhythm and fluency poor
Excites when caregiver approaches			Pre-verbal turn-taking Uses proto- words	Requests assistance in handling objects	Volume, pitch control poor
Wary of strangers, unfamiliar situations				Hi and bye initiates topics nonverbally and vocally	Uses: I, me, you, my, mine Simple topic control
Quiets when being held				Demonstrates sympathy, empathy, and sharing nonverbally	Interruptions are common, but occur at syntactic junctures or in response prosodic cues

Months 24–36	Months 36–48	Months 48–60	Months 60+	Year 6
Answers questions	Understands much of what is said	Most vowels and diphthongs	Indirect requests	State of problem
Follows two step commands	Role playing	Make believe	Uses deictic terms: this, that, here, there	Communicate facts about world to friends and family
Some plurals, past tense	Uses: okay, uh, huh as fillers	Well formed sentences		
Uses: in, or, under	Code switching (simpler language to younger child or doll)	Story structure	Uses variety of questions: where, when, why, how many, what do you do	Uses contingent queries
Knows chief body parts Verbs predominate		100% intelligible		
Relates own experiences		Repeats four digits		Describes functions of objects
Can reason out answers to questions	Request permission	Repeats word of four syllables	Extends topic	
Can give name, gender, age	Begins make believe	Animal names	Uses of descriptive terms (adjectives and adverbs)	Tells complete stories
50% intelligible	Corrects others	Uses: over and under		Meta-pragmatic awareness
Three+ word sentences	Beginning of checks on background information	Uses: four prepositions such as over and under	Knows opposites (big-little, hard-soft, heavy-light)	Use of anaphora
What questions	Uses: why questions	Names objects in pictures	Counts to ten	Conforms to Gricean conver-sational postulates
900–1000 word vocabulary		One or more colors	Speech entirely intelligible despite faulty articulation	
Short dialogs	75% intelligible	Verbalization accompanies activities		Understands and uses some idioms
Topic intro and changes topic	Masters m, h, y, n, w, d, p, and h	Follow commands when objects are not in sight	All vowels and consonants	
Expresses emotions	Uses indirection	Rapid topic shifts	Repeats sentences as long as nine words	
Clarifications and requests clarifications	Terminates conversation appropriately	Topic continuity over five turns	Defines common object	
Heaps and sequences as proto-narratives	Primitive narratives	Turn-taking repairs	Follows three commands	
Turn pauses about twice duration of adults	Topic maintenance over three turns		Knows simple time concepts – morning, night, day, tomorrow, yesterday, today, later	
Repetition common as topic maintenance strategy	Uses modals (would, could, can, etc.)			
Responds to repair sequences initiated by adults	Uses past tense		Long sentences, compound and some complex	
	Uses pauses as a cue for initiating turn-taking		Provides assistance, altruism	
Some speech adaptation to different listeners	Anticipates next turn at talk			
	Some completion of other speakers' thoughts		Asks for permission	
Uses some politeness formulas Violates turn-taking 5% of the time	Infers background information from stories			

prototypes. For example, Johnny's manner of pragmatic engagement in the ritualistic greeting could be described as falling well toward the dominant pole, as somewhat impolite-indeferent and as somewhat asynchronous-unresponsive (eg, did not synchronize topics or length of turn-taking in terms of the social framework provided in a greeting) to his co-communicators. Timothy William Smith's pragmatic engagement in the ritualistic greeting could be described as falling toward the incommunicative pole, however, as somewhat irrelevant-verbose and asynchronous-unresponsive but also as somewhat too expository-pedantic.

Both the number of moments included in the circle and the number of prototypes within each of the 12 manners of engagement could be expanded to provide a more fine-grained description of a child's or adolescent's characteristic manner of pragmatic engagement. Note, however, that even this simplified figure suggests ways to characterize the typical pragmatic manner of engagement associated with different types of childhood psychopathology. For example, children with ADHD and ODD often engage in discourse in ways that are best described by the two moments that are nearest the dominant pole (assertive-quarrelsome-belligerent and impolite-indeferent-rude) plus the two moments that contain admixtures of dominance and incommunicativeness (asynchronous-unresponsive-monologic and irrelevant-verbose-rambling). In addition, some children with ADHD-ODD also have prosody problems (eg, loudness and speech rate). Similarly, children who are high functioning but fall along the autistic spectrum often engage in discourse in ways that are best described by the two moments surrounding the incommunicable pole (irrelevant-verbose-rambling and aprosodic-agrammatic-unintelligible) plus the moment between the dominant and incommunicable poles (asynchronous-unresponsive-monologic) and the moment between the dominant and communicable pole (literal-expository-pedantic) and its complement (nonliteral-fictional-poetic).

One of the most important tasks in assessing a child's pragmatic competence is to evaluate the use of whatever linguistic and gestural behaviors they have developed in relation to the specific contexts of interaction and event frames that figure importantly in their social, familial, and educational daily life. The dimensions that are important to consider when making such assessments concern whether the child's communication is appropriate, legitimate, normative, effective, and sincere. Each of these sociocultural dimensions seems to be continuous, with communicative behaviors falling between antipodes of clearly acceptable and clearly unacceptable communicative behavior. Coupled with the assessment of the emergence and adequacy and well-formedness of the communication (eg, a child can attempt to tell a narrative of his or her experience that fails to order events sequentially and causally and is too vague to interpret even though the attempt is appropriate, legitimate, normative, and sincere within the communication context), use of these dimensions can provide information about the child's ability to communicate in a socially acceptable and effective manner.

Formal assessment of a child's pragmatic abilities typically includes observation; collection of checklists from parents and teachers, if applicable; and formal tests. Two checklists that provide norm-referenced or criterion-referenced scores for English-speaking children in the United States seem to be quite useful in assessing a child's pragmatic language competence and other aspects of social relatedness and adjustment: the Children's Communication Checklist–2 [14] for children between ages 4 and 16.11, and the Pragmatic Profile for children between ages 5 and 21.11 provided in the Comprehensive Evaluation of Language Fundamentals–4 [19]. These checklists provide information about various domains of pragmatic language competence, such as use and comprehension of nonverbal communicative behaviors; ability to initiate and respond to conversational requests; ability to use context; ability to initiate, sustain, and switch topics appropriately; and information about a child's speech, syntactic, and semantic development. The Children's Communication Checklist–2 also provides an index that is "helpful in identifying children with a communicative profile that might be characteristic of language impairment or ASD [autistic spectrum disorder]" [36]. Both of these checklists are relatively easy to score and can be used in conjunction with parent and child interviews to ascertain if a referral to a speech pathologist is advisable for further assessment and treatment. It is likely that the speech pathologist will use both formal testing procedures and controlled participant observation during their examination as part of their diagnostic work-up. Results of such a work-up pinpoint the main features of a child's pragmatic impairment and formulate a treatment plan to help remedy them. Often, pragmatic skill training and language-speech therapy are recommended.

Pragmatic language competence and psychiatric comorbidities

Because formal assessment of the structural features of language and their development have been available for quite some time, more is known about the extent to which specific language impairment or expressive-receptive language disorders are comorbid with psychiatric disorders (see article on language impairment and psychiatric comorbidities by Im-Bolten and Cohen in this issue for review) than about the comorbidity of pragmatic language impairments and psychiatric disorders. Over the past 10 years, however, strong empirical evidence has established that deficits in pragmatic language skill are associated with, or a constituent of, many developmental and psychiatric conditions and contribute significantly to functional impairments in school, in peer relationships, and in psychiatric adjustment [37]. For example, impairments in pragmatic competence are considered a constitutive feature of developmental disorders falling along the autistic spectrum (pervasive developmental disorder, not otherwise specified, autism, and Asperger's syndrome) [38–41]. Interestingly, many of these children do not evidence impairments or only minor impairments in their structural language competencies

[16,42,43]. These children can do very well on formal tests of syntax, for example, but fail to formulate an effective and appropriate request to be included in ongoing peer interaction or gaming or abide by the most simple relevance stipulations (eg, as when they provide much more information about a topic of their interest than is required to sustain a conversation).

Impairments in pragmatic competence are also evident in many children with ADHD, ODD, and conduct disorder. The overall degree of impairment in pragmatic functioning of children with ADHD has been reported to be as severe as high-functioning children along the autistic spectrum [44]. The pragmatic competence of children with ADHD is reliably and repeated found to be worse than typically developing peers [45]. These findings also emerge when comparing children with ODD and conduct disorder with typically developing controls [46]. In fact, in the study by Gilmour and colleagues [46], greater than two thirds of the children with conduct disorder also exhibited impairment in the pragmatic competencies. Future research is needed to explore if the types of pragmatic difficulties that children with different externalizing disorders experience are similar to each other or vary across pragmatic domains. There is also evidence that children with internalizing disorders also have pragmatic impairments [47], and these seem to be different than those exhibited by children with externalizing disorders.

What is emerging from recent research and longstanding clinical observation is that children with psychiatric disorders are at a high risk for having or developing impairments in their pragmatic communicative competence, and these impairments can be as severe and as functionally maladaptive as those often exhibited by children with structural language disorders. Unfortunately, there is little research on the efficacy or effectiveness of treatments focused on improving impairments in pragmatic communicative competence [48–50]. It is hoped that the contemporary attempt to improve pragmatic assessment instruments and the growing awareness of the impact of pragmatic deficits on children's social, interpersonal, and school functioning result in the identification of validated targets for intervention. Currently, numerous social skill training-like treatments, conducted in groups or less often individually, seem to remediate children's general level of pragmatic functioning as assessed clinically and observationally.

Although impairments in pragmatic communicative competence are described and recognized as disorders by speech and language pathologists, they are not now nor have they been in the past considered a disorder in the *Diagnostic and Statistical Manual*. Discussion over whether they should be considered as a separate type of developmental language disorder continues and it is hoped will be clarified when new diagnostic instruments are used in epidemiologic and developmental psychopathologic studies. Among the set of questions that need to be answered are the following: Are deficits in pragmatic communication competence a consequence of, a defining symptom of, or a frequent comorbidity with particular psychiatric disorders; or, are at least some of the symptoms that define particular psychiatric disorders consequences or defining symptoms of pragmatic communicative impairments? It is entirely possible that, for example, the turn-taking and topic control impairments that are noted in the *Diagnostic and Statistical Manual-IV* symptom list for ADHD are either the same as or different from the turn-taking and topic control impairments that children without ADHD exhibit as part of their pragmatic problems, at both the surface level and at the etiologic level. Unfortunately, too little is known about the cause of both ADHD and pragmatic language disorders to answer these questions with confidence.

Genetics and neurobiology of pragmatic language competence

Less in known about the genetics and neurobiology of pragmatic language competence than about reading and language generally. There is some evidence that pragmatic language disorders aggregate in families, although this evidence is not based on replicated studies [51]. In so far as there seems to be a strong comorbidity between structural language disorders (expressive-receptive language disorders) and pragmatic impairments, future research is need to decipher if patterns of inheritance are similar for the types of impairments or distinct [52]. Because pragmatic language competence requires social competence and social inference abilities, whereas on the standard view structural language competence does not, there is good reason to expect differences in the way the disorders segregate and what combination of genetic abnormalities may play significant etiologic roles in the two disorders.

Brain areas involved in different facets of pragmatic language skill have been identified tentatively on the basis of studies of the consequences of traumatic brain injury, on MRI and fMRI descriptive and experimental research. Much of the research is constrained by technical limitations in the use of imaging techniques with young children (eg, the use of sedation, and for fMRI, long periods of restrictive movement). Further, it may be unreasonable to assume that the underlying neurobiologic organization of pragmatic skills found in pragmatically impaired adults, who are likely implementing compensatory strategies for pragmatic tasks, is similar to those in children who are developing pragmatic skills or unable yet to compensate for impairments. In addition, many of the key pragmatic domains of interest are difficult to capture in experimental paradigms suitable for imaging (eg, conversational discourse, turn-taking, story telling). There is evidence that overall pragmatic abilities are more adversely affected with right than left hemisphere damage, particularly for extralinguistic domains (eg, gesturing), but more refined research promises to specify differential neurocircuitry for differing pragmatic impairments [53].

Some advances have been made in characterizing brain areas involved in different aspects of pragmatic tasks. For example, the superior temporal gyrus is involved in prosody processing bilaterally in adults and children.

Children also show right lateralization in the middle frontal gyrus. Activation of brain areas depends on the tasks the subjects are asked to complete, but even quite narrowly focused tasks have revealed how different brain areas are activated when processing subtle prosodic differences in utterances. For example, in a study using functional echo planar imaging, subjects were asked to make judgments about three kinds of utterances: (1) questions in the form of statements with rising intonation, (2) statements with falling intonation, and (3) questions with falling intonation plus the typical word order change. Increased activation in bilateral inferior frontal and temporal regions occurred with questions in the form of statements with rising intonation over the other two kinds of utterances [54]. As the authors conclude, differential brain activation indicates that regions of the brain are responsive "to intonationally marked illocutionary differences between questions and statements" [54]. Prosodic cues that seem to have emotional significance, such as the variability in the spectral properties of a speech signal, have often been associated with right hemisphere processing and seem to be impaired in patients with right hemisphere brain damage, whereas prosodic cues associated with linguistic significance have been found to be left lateralized and associated with left hemisphere damage. In general, the evidence suggests that the neural substrates for pragmatic, syntactic, and semantic processing are both similar and distinct, with bilateral involvement of superior temporal regions for pragmatic and semantic but not syntactic processing, and left inferior temporal-fusiform involvement across all three types of processing [55]. Prosodic impairments are especially important in understanding pragmatic competence, however, because children with these impairments are often rated as having lowered social communication abilities. For example, children who use inappropriate sentential stress and hypernasality seem to have less social and communicative skill than those who do not.

The ability to understand and convey conversational implicatures, verbal and nonverbal, is central to attaining pragmatic competence. Implicatures of utterances are unstated circumstances that are held to be true in the communication context and which often clarify surface oddities of utterances in the context of an exchange. For example, if one is asked to read *Harry Potter and the Sorcerer's Stone*, and one responds "I saw the movie," it is assumed that this answer is indeed relevant to answering the question, is informative enough to answer the question, answers the question in a truthful way, and is an orderly rather than obscure or obfuscating answer. This answer conveys, in context, that one did not read the book but saw the movie. Implicatures can vary in the degree to which inferencing is needed for comprehension. Adults with either left or right hemisphere brain damage seem to have more difficulty interpreting implicatures than their normal counterparts [56].

Like implicatures, understanding sarcasm, irony, and lying requires a level of inferencing that understanding simple, literal utterances does not require.

To understand sarcasm, irony, and lying requires inferences about intentions and about knowledge about one's knowledge of the state of affairs in question. Those neural substrates activated when attempting these more complicated pragmatic communications overlap with those involved in theory of mind tasks, executive function tasks, and empathy tasks. Prefrontal regions figure prominently in understanding the latter tasks and are also involved in understanding sarcasm. It has been suggested that the right frontal lobe mediates the understanding of sarcasm by integrating affective processing with the perspective taking necessary in theory of mind tasks [57].

Imaging of the brain during story telling and comprehension (eg, in understanding the gist of a story) or when trying to make sense of topic changes versus reasoning in discourse is arguably in its infancy. From the few studies available, a general finding is that there are more brain areas involved in these pragmatic tasks than had once been thought and the theory that speech functions are left lateralized may need significant revision. For example, whereas a left hemisphere bias involving Broca's and Wernicke's areas is evident when making sense (identifying the gist) of a conversation, they are augmented by their right homologs, right dorsolateral prefrontal cortex, and the cerebellum when appraising topic changes in discourse [58]. Similarly, when studying discourse generation, there is bilateral activation of the cerebral hemispheres that progresses to left-lateralized activation, a model quite distinct from the left hemisphere dominant model.

Summary

Pragmatic competence involves the synergistic use of linguistic and social-cultural knowledge to produce utterances in context that are effective and appropriate. A growing number of research studies implicate pragmatic impairments as a key feature, not just of autistic spectrum disorders, but also of externalizing and internalizing disorders. Pragmatic impairments have functional consequences for children ranging from difficulties with peer acceptance, friendship building, and maintenance, to predisposing children to develop psychiatric problems. For these reasons, pediatricians and other health care workers must become more sensitive to identifying pragmatic communicative impairments as soon as is feasible.

In this article, a number of different tools have been provided to assist in the recognition of the various domains comprising pragmatic language competence, a rough sketch of the order in which pragmatic skills develop, and a brief sample of some of the research characterizing the neurobiologic substrates involved in different aspects of pragmatic skill. Several vignettes were provided to indicate just how useful an appraisal of a child's discourse participation can be in formulating hypotheses about the child's developmental level and psychiatric problems. In addition, several instruments were recommended that can help the pediatrician assess a child's pragmatic language abilities. It is hoped that current and future research will produce more and better pragmatic assessment instruments and detail interventions that have been shown to be both efficacious and effective for precisely defined pragmatic communication problems.

References

[1] Levinson SC. Pragmatics. Cambridge (UK): Cambridge University Press; 1983.
[2] Hymes D. Foundations in sociolinguistics: an ethnographic approach. Philadelphia: University of Pennsylvania Press; 1974.
[3] Ochs E, editor. Developmental pragmatics. New York: Academic Press; 1979.
[4] Bara BG, Bosco FM, Bucciarelli M. Developmental pragmatics in normal and abnormal children. Brain Lang 1999;68:507–28.
[5] Ninio A, Snow CE. Pragmatic development: essays in developmental science. In: Kagan J, editor. Boulder (CO): Westview Press, Inc.; 1996.
[6] Ninio A, Snow CE. The development of pragmatics: learning to use language appropriately. In: Handbook of child language acquisition. San Diego (CA): Academic Press; 1999. p. 347–83.
[7] Leinonen E, Letts C, Smith BR. Children's pragmatic communication difficulties. London: Whurr Publishers Ltd.; 2000.
[8] Sperber D, Wilson D. Pragmatics, modularity and mind-reading. Mind & Language 2002; 17:3–23.
[9] Searle JR. Speech acts: an essay in the philosophy of language. London: Cambridge University Press; 1969.
[10] Austin J. How to do things with words. Oxford (UK): Clarendon Press; 1962.
[11] Burke K. A grammar of motives. New York: Prentice-Hall; 1945.
[12] Burke K. Language as symbolic action. Berkeley (CA): University of California Press; 1969.
[13] Sperber D, Wilson D. Relevance: communication and cognition. Cambridge (UK): Harvard University Press; 1986.
[14] Bishop DVM. The children's communication checklist, 2nd edition. London: The Psychological Corporation Limited; 2003.
[15] Adams C. Practitioner review: the assessment of language pragmatics. J Child Psychol Psychiatry 2002;43:973–87.
[16] Bishop DVM. Pragmatic language impairment: a correlate of SLI, a distinct subgroup, or part of the autistic continuum? In: Bishop DVM, Leonard L, editors. Specific language impairments in children: causes, characteristics, intervention, and outcome. Hove (UK): Psychology Press; 2000. p. 99–113.
[17] Rice ML, Sell MA, Hadley PA. The social interactive coding system (SICS): an on-line, clinically relevant descriptive tool. Language, Speech & Hearing Services in the Schools 1990;21: 2–14.
[18] Carrow-Woolfolk E. Comprehensive assessment of spoken language. Circle Pines (MN): American Guidance Service; 1999.
[19] Semel E, Wiig EH, Secord WA. Clinical evaluation of language fundamentals. 4th edition. San Antonio (TX): The Psychological Corporation; 2003.
[20] Phelps-Terasaki D, Phelps-Gunn T. Test of pragmatic language. Los Angeles (CA): Western Psychological Services; 1992.
[21] Adams C, Cooke R, Crutchley A, et al. Assessment of comprehension and expression 6-11. Windsor (UK): Nfer-Nelson Publishing Company Ltd.; 2001.
[22] Wiig EH, Secord WA. Test of language competence–expanded edition. San Antonio (TX): The Psychological Corporation, Harcourt Brace Jovanovich, Inc.; 1988.

[23] Wiig E. Criterion referenced inventory of language. San Antonio (TX): The Psychological Corporation Harcourt Brace Jovanovich, Inc.; 1990.

[24] Bishop D. Expression, reception, and recall of narrative instrument. London: Harcourt Assessment; 2004.

[25] Adams C, Bishop DVM. Conversational characteristics of children with semantic-pragmatic disorder. I: Exchange structure, turntaking, repairs and cohesion. Br J Disord Commun 1989;24:211–39.

[26] Bowers L, Barrett M, Huisingh R, et al. Test of problem solving–revised. East Moline (IL): LinguiSystems; 1994.

[27] Seymour HN, Roeper TW, de Villiers J. Diagnostic evaluation of language variation, in DELV (criterion referenced). San Antonio (TX): The Psychological Corporation, Harcourt Assessment Company; 2003.

[28] Rinaldi W. Understanding ambiguity: an assessment of pragmatic meaning comprehension. London: NferNelson Publishing Company Ltd.; 1996.

[29] Bishop DVM, Adams C. Conversational characteristics of children with semantic-pragmatic disorder. II: What features lead to a judgement of inappropriacy? Br J Disord Commun 1989;24:241–63.

[30] Russell RL, Grizzle K, Shabazian I. Pragmatic language disorders: assessing the assessments. Presented at the Wisconsin Speech-Language Pathology & Audiology Association. Madison (WI), April 16, 2005.

[31] American Speech Language Hearing Association. Pragmatics, socially speaking. 1997–2006. Available at: http://www.nsslha.org/public/speech/development/pragmatics.htm. Accessed December 14, 2006.

[32] American Speech Language Hearing Association. Pragmatic language tips. 1997–2006. Available at: http://www.nsslha.org/public/speech/development/Pragmatic-Language-Tips.htm. Accessed December 14, 2006.

[33] Child Development Institute LLC. Language development chart. 1998–2006, Available at: http://childdevelopmentinfo.com/development/language_development.shtml. Accessed January 23, 2007.

[34] Feldman HM. Evaluation and management of language and speech disorders in preschool children. Pediatr Rev 2005;26:131–41.

[35] Parent-Child Services Group Inc. Pragmatic language development. Available at: http://www.parent-childservices.com/handouts/pragmatic_language_development.htm. Accessed December 14, 2006.

[36] Bishop DVM. Children's communication checklist-2. United States edition. San Antonio (TX): Harcourt Assessment, Inc.; 2006.

[37] Grizzle KL, Russell RL. Language disorders and psychiatric comorbitiy: a meta-analytic study. Presented at the 9th European Congress of Psychology. Granada (Spain), July 2005.

[38] Tager-Flusberg H. What language reveals about the understanding of minds in children with autism. In: Baron-Cohen S, Tager-Flusberg H, Cohen DJ, editors. Understanding other minds. Oxford (UK): Oxford University Press; 1993. p. 138–57.

[39] Mawhood L, Howlin P, Rutter M. Autism and developmental receptive language disorder: a comparative follow-up in early adult life. I: Cognitive and language outcomes. J Child Psychol Psychiatry 2000;41:547–59.

[40] Lord C. The complexity of social behaviour in autism. In: Baron-Cohen S, Tager-Flusberg H, Cohen DJ, editors. Understanding other minds: perspectives from autism. Oxford (UK): Oxford University Press; 1993. p. 643–55.

[41] Rapin I. Practitioner review: developmental language disorders: a clinical update. J Child Psychol Psychiatry 1996;37:643–55.

[42] Norbury CF, Nash M, Baird G, et al. Using a parental checklist to identify diagnostic groups in children with communication impairment: a validation of the Children's Communication Checklist-2. Int J Lang Commun Disord 2004;39:345–64.

[43] Barrett S, Prior M, Manjiviona J. Children on the borderlands of autism. Autism 2004;8: 61–87.

[44] Bishop DVM, Baird G. Parent and teacher report of pragmatic aspects of communication: use of the Children's Communication Checklist in a clinical setting. Dev Med Child Neurol 2001;43:809–18.

[45] Geurts HM, Verte S, Oosterlaan J, et al. Can the Children's Communication Checklist differentiate between children with autism, children with ADHD, and normal controls? J Child Psychol Psychiatry 2004;45:1437–53.

[46] Gilmour J, Hill B, Place M, et al. Social communication deficits in conduct disorder: a clinical and community survey. J Child Psychol Psychiatry 2004;45:967–78.

[47] Tse WS, Bond AJ. The impact of depression on social skills. J Nerv Ment Dis 2004;192: 260–8.

[48] Adams C. Clinical diagnostic and intervention studies of children with semantic-pragmatic language disorder. Int J Lang Commun Disord 2001;36:289–305.

[49] Hyter YD, Rogers-Adkinson DL, Self TL, et al. Pragmatic language intervention for children with language and emotional/behavioral disorders. Communication Disorders Quarterly 2001;23:4–16.

[50] Penn C. Pragmatic assessment and therapy for persons with brain damage: what have clinicians gleaned in two decades? Brain Lang 1999;68:535–52.

[51] Bishop DV, Laws G, Adams C, et al. High heritability of speech and language impairments in 6-year-old twins demonstrated using parent and teacher report. Behav Genet 2006;36: 173–84.

[52] Bishop DVM. Genetic influences on language impairment and literacy problems in children: same or different? J Child Psychol Psychiatry 2001;42:189–98.

[53] Cutica I, Bucciarelli M, Bara BG. Neuropragmatics: extralinguistic pragmatic ability is better preserved in left-hemisphere-damaged patients than in right-hemisphere-damaged patients. Brain Lang 2006;98:12–25.

[54] Doherty CP, West WC, Dilley LC, et al. Question/statement judgments: an fMRI study of intonation processing. Hum Brain Mapp 2004;23:85–98.

[55] Kuperberg GR, McGuire PK, Bullmore ET, et al. Common and distinct neural substrates for pragmatic, semantic, and syntactic processing of spoken sentences: an fMRI study. J Cogn Neurosci 2000;12:321–41.

[56] Kasher A, Batori G, Soroker N, et al. Effects of right- and left-hemisphere damage on understanding conversational implicatures. Brain Lang 1999;68:566–90.

[57] Shamay-Tsoory SG, Tomer R, Aharon-Peretz J. The neuroanatomical basis of understanding sarcasm and its relationship to social cognition. Neuropsychology 2005;19:288–300.

[58] Caplan R, Dapretto M. Making sense during conversation: an fMRI study. Neuroreport 2001;12:3625–32.

ELSEVIER
SAUNDERS

PEDIATRIC CLINICS
OF NORTH AMERICA

Pediatr Clin N Am 54 (2007) 507–523

Developmental Dyslexia

Kenneth L. Grizzle, PhD

*Department of Pediatrics, Medical College of Wisconsin, Children's Hospital of Wisconsin,
8701 Watertown Plank Road, Wauwatosa, WI 53226, USA*

Problems learning to read potentially are multifaceted. Broadly, deficits can fall into one or more of the following areas: difficulty reading whole words accurately and eventually reading them fluently in context; cognitive, language, and vocabulary deficits that limit children's ability to derive meaning from books; and lack of motivation [1]. These three areas not necessarily are independent; a loss of interest in and motivation to read may be the consequence of difficulties in reading or language processing. Within each of these areas are additional processes that may break down and contribute to deficient reading skills.

Lyon and colleagues [2] define dyslexia as "characterized by difficulties with accurate and/or fluent word recognition and by poor spelling and decoding abilities." These difficulties are unexpected in relation to other cognitive skills and occur despite effective reading instruction. This generally agreed-on definition suggests that individuals who have dyslexia show deficits in the most basic of reading processes, word decoding, which can limit comprehension of material read. Decoding is the process of applying phonetic principals to sound words out. Reading requires children to appreciate that words are composed of symbols and sounds. Once children understand that each letter and many letter combinations have sounds and are worth discriminating from one another, they have attained the alphabetic principal [3], a prerequisite to developing effective word reading skills. Children who struggle to develop the alphabetic principal likely find it difficult to establish decoding skills and find the process of learning to read a challenge. Simply put, dyslexia is a specific reading disorder characterized by deficits in word reading or reading fluency.

Normal reading development

Appreciating the typical developmental process of reading is helpful to a better understanding of areas that might contribute to reading difficulties

---

E-mail address: kgrizzle@mcw.edu

0031-3955/07/$ - see front matter © 2007 Published by Elsevier Inc.
doi:10.1016/j.pcl.2007.02.015

in children. Behaviorally, children often become familiar with books at the end of their first year of life through grabbing and mouthing them. As children progress through toddlerhood, they appreciate phrasing and intonation patterns used by caregivers when being read to. Toddlers who are read to consistently identify book illustrations and engage in dialog with their caregivers about the content of the written word; children may memorize words and phrases in sections of frequently read books. When asked to pick out a particular book, children at this age often are able to do so as if they are reading the title. It is not unusual for preschool-aged children to "read" books as they sit on the floor, opening books and rehearsing memorized text, even turning pages at appropriate times. During this period, children begin to recognize print as distinct from scribble and even "write" in a meaningful way. The ability to use symbols (scribbling) reflects children's entrée into the abstract nature of language, oral and written. These early literacy activities are reflected and encouraged best through play.

As children enter formal school settings, they transition from prereading skills to a stage referred to as "phonetic cue reading" [1]. During this period, children systematically begin to associate the orthographic representation of letters with their associated sounds. At this point, however, children are not mapping sounds onto all letters in a word, but only on select letter strings, notably the beginning and ending letters, such as the /b/ and /l/ sounds in ball. To become effective readers, children must progress to the point of recognizing all letters within a word and mapping orthographic representations on the correct phoneme. Children who are in the early stages of developing reading skills exert considerable effort in their attempts to decode words. Each word they encounter may be considered novel and require detective work to read accurately. Only with repeated exposure, reading words in context, can words be transferred into children's automatic lexicon. It is at this point that reading fluency and speed begin developing.

Language and reading

Language contributes to the development of reading skills on several levels. Two comprehensive reviews of the early reading literature conclude that oral language development plays a critical role in learning to read [1,4]. Intuitively, and perhaps having received the most empiric support, is the strong relationship between oral language skills (including vocabulary) and reading comprehension [5,6]. Vocabulary, however, also plays a role in the development of decoding skills and phonologic sensitivity [7,8].

Phonologic sensitivity—children's ability to identify and manipulate sounds in words—is a microlevel language skill compared with syntactic and semantic processes. There is agreement that the development of this skill is crucial to the acquisition of word decoding skills. Early manifestations of phonologic sensitivity (often referred to as phonemic awareness) in toddlers and preschoolers include the recognition of rhyming words (ball rhymes with hall). Typically developing children at this age also often recognize other large phonologic segments, such as syllables, and develop an awareness of alliteration ("Bill's blue ball was bouncy"). It is not until approximately 5 years of age that children typically are able to develop phonologic sensitivity at a phoneme level [9].

As children enter and progress through kindergarten, the single best predictor of later reading skills is alphabet recognition [10]. Identification of letters is a better predictor of reading skill acquisition than letter-sound understanding [11]. It seems, however, that learning letter names alone has little direct benefit on reading development; rather, it affects children's ability to learn the corresponding sounds associated with the letter [9].

Children who are developing phonologic sensitivity and an appreciation for English orthography and whose syntactic and semantic language structures are intact are in a good position to develop strong word reading and decoding skills.

Reading comprehension

During the primary grades, learning to read is defined as learning to recognize and decode words. At this point, reading comprehension is constrained largely by limited print word awareness. As decoding and word recognition skills improve, there are other factors that play a critical role in children's ability to derive meaning from written text, including vocabulary, oral comprehension, and working memory [12]. Children use multiple metacognitive approaches to help with understanding text. Children need to understand the structure of reading material, which varies with type of text (ie, narrative or expository) [13]. Having an understanding of story structure influences how one reads, interprets, and ultimately understands a piece of literature. The same can be said for how individuals approach a textbook (expository text); that is, the cognitive schemata for a particular subject influences the author and the reader. Readers also use various strategies to enhance comprehension. Examples of studied strategies used frequently include goal setting, inference making, identifying the main idea, summarizing, predicting, monitoring, and backtracking [13].

Children grow up in families with varying levels of literacy and social interaction. Evidence to date suggests that the home literacy environment predicts kindergarten literacy skills modestly to strongly [1,14]. Family influences on reading development tend to fall into five areas: value placed on literacy as reflected by parent reading and encouraging their children to read; press for achievement, including expectations for children to achieve and responding to children's interest in reading; availability of reading material within the home; reading to and with children; and opportunities for verbal interaction [15]. The last area speaks to the value of parent-child interactions and its affect, most notably, on vocabulary development, an area known to be an important component of reading comprehension.

Developmental progression of dyslexia

Although much is written about early predictors of reading problems, the majority of research has focused on reading broadly rather than dyslexia specifically. The connection between early and persistent language deficits and reading is well established. There are early red flags that suggest children are at increased risk for decoding deficits. Schatschneider and Torgeson [16] recently outlined the developmental progression of this disorder, suggesting that children's poor understanding of the alphabetic principal late in kindergarten or in first grade makes it difficult for them to read unfamiliar words (at this point in their life), even though the words may be part of their oral vocabulary. Even before attempts are made to decode words, children must be able to recognize letters of the alphabet. At this age, children's ability to identify letters of the alphabet randomly is a better predictor of later reading difficulties than an entire battery of tests [1]. Results of a large district-wide sample of children [17] suggest that if kindergarten children falling in the bottom 25th percentile of letter naming are identified as at risk, nearly 80% can be identified accurately as having a reading disorder in first grade and only 10% would be missed.

Moving from letter recognition to sound-symbol correspondence requires the ability to map the orthographic properties of the letter on sound properties. Children who have dyslexia struggle with these tasks, which results in their reading slowly, attempting to apply phonetic decoding skills to most words, making frequent errors when reading, and all too often avoiding the reading process because they find it frustrating and difficult. After mastering the alphabetic principal, most children begin to apply phonetic decoding skills effectively and proceed (discussed previously) to frequent reading, which increases sight word vocabulary and in turn fluency. Poor word decoding skills together with few sight words have a negative impact on children's ability to read text fluently. For children who are dyslexic, their poor lower-level skills (phonologic processing and word decoding) create a bottleneck in their academic progress. Impaired reading has an impact on their ability to tap into broad general knowledge. With limited access to text, children, adolescents, and adults who are dyslexic are at risk for having an unfair ceiling placed on their access to knowledge. Stanovich [18] coined the phrase, "Matthew effect," referring to the impact dyslexia can have on individuals. In essence, individuals who can read do read and benefit from doing so. Conversely, individuals who are dyslexic read considerably less than typically developing peers, which affects their continued development of reading skills, vocabulary, and general knowledge. Large-scale longitudinal studies identify increasing cognitive disparities between strong and poor readers [19,20].

Comorbidities

The co-occurrence of other psychiatric conditions and developmental disorders in individuals who have a reading disability (RD) is high. One study of disorders co-occurring with a RD included a sample of 179 children; more than half (52%) of the children who had a reading disorder had additional diagnoses [21]. The frequency of overlap between dyslexia and other developmental and psychiatric conditions warrants discussion.

Cognitive

Language functioning
The connection between language and reading is clear and well supported. As discussed previously, phonologic processing has a direct causal link to early reading (decoding and word reading) skills; children who have strong phonologic awareness are likely to develop strong word decoding skills and those who have poor phonologic awareness are at much greater risk for being poor word decoders [22–24].The relationship between oral language comprehension and vocabulary development and word decoding, however, is less apparent. In an informative study from the United Kingdom, Snowling and colleagues followed a group of children identified as having speech or language impairment from preschool through adolescence. Literacy (reading and spelling) measures were administered at 5.5, 8, and 15 years of age. Although elevated relative to the expected population rate (3%–5%), children who had impaired language had rates of word reading (8%) and reading comprehension (12%) difficulties that were not as high as expected [25]. Further, children who had phonologic disorders resolved at 5.5 were at no greater risk for literacy or language difficulties. This picture changes as children enter adolescence. Adolescents who have preschool language impairment, resolved or not, showed significantly greater rates of word reading and reading comprehension deficits than normal controls. The rate of word reading deficits rose to 49%, and reading comprehension deficits greater than 1 SD lower than the mean increased to 54% [26]. Nonverbal cognitive functioning did not explain these changes entirely.

This set of studies provides evidence for a concept Scarborough [27] refers to as a period of "illusory recovery." Children who have early language deficits resolved by school entry seem to progress nicely with early literacy skills. In the absence of phonologic processing deficits, these children are able to develop word reading and decoding skills in a manner similar to same-age peers. As they progress through the grades and the language demands, oral and written, change dramatically, however, children who have early language delays not only lack the language-processing skills, impairing reading comprehension further, but also their early deficits bleed into their ability to decode words effectively [12,26].

The relevance of this phenomenon to dyslexia is seen in the evaluation and diagnosis of reading problems in adolescents and young adults. Dyslexia is considered a developmental disorder, although evidence suggests the need to obtain a thorough speech and language history from middle school– and high school–aged children presenting with reading problems.

What may seem to be late-appearing, word-reading deficits may be a residual language disorder.

Matthew effect

Less a comorbidity and more a correlate of poor reading skills is the concept referred to by Stanovich [18] as the Matthew effect. The idea behind this concept is the boot-strapping effect of early literacy skills: individuals who have strong phonologic processing (and general language) skills likely develop the alphabetic principal and, in turn, strong word attack skills. The ability to read begets an interest in reading, which translates into a greater likelihood to engage in literacy activities [19,20]. There is evidence that reading (or avoiding reading) has a reciprocal effect on basic reading skills (phonologic processing, decoding skills, fluency, and so forth) [28] and several cognitive processes, including children who have dyslexia showing a slight drop in verbal cognitive functioning over time [29] and having smaller vocabularies [28], which have a further impact on reading comprehension.

Motor functioning

The occurrence of motor problems in children who are dyslexic is not surprising in light of the identified involvement of cerebellar functioning in this population [30,31]. There is evidence that the motor problems typically associated with attention-deficit/hyperactivity disorder (ADHD) may be mediated by RD [32]. Motor deficits seem to be global in nature, encompassing fine and gross motor impairments [32,33]. There is some question about the severity of these deficits; Kooistra and colleagues [32] and Iversen and colleagues [33] suggest that impairment is severe enough to warrant a diagnosis of developmental coordination disorder and referral for a motor evaluation. Review of the data reported by Kooistra and colleagues [32], however, finds that groups of children who had RD had average scores on the Bruininks-Oseretsky Test of Motor Proficiency [34] and the Developmental Test of Visual-Motor Integration [35], although significantly different from controls. Further, scores of less than a single SD were considered by the investigators to be at or below the cut-off range for clinical significance. Iversen and colleagues [33], alternatively, found that greater than 50% of children who have RD have motor coordination problems (manual dexterity and balance) that place them at or below the fifth percentile.

In sum, the evidence to date suggests a link between motor impairment and dyslexia; at the least, children who have RD are at greater risk for having minor impairment in fine and gross motor skills. The question of whether or not this level of impairment has a functional impact on these children, and in turn warrants comprehensive motor evaluations, is not clear. This requires evaluation by astute clinicians who are aware of the potential relationship between reading and motor problems to screen for deficits and make appropriate referrals when necessary. One potential area for functional impact is graphomotor skills. Berninger and colleagues [36–38] have provided considerable evidence of the potentially negative impact graphomotor deficits can have on written output, including development of written expression skills. They provide additional evidence indicating that early and intensive intervention can minimize the effects of motor impairment on written output [33,38,39].

Psychosocial

The relationship between reading problems and psychiatric status, most notably disruptive behavior disorders, is well established [40–43]. A recent nationwide study in the United Kingdom found the odds ratios for the psychiatric conditions ADHD, conduct disorder, anxiety, and depression in children who have RD range from 1.04 (depression) to 3.82 (ADHD); all but depression were statistically significant. Despite high risk ratios, however, a small minority of children met diagnostic criteria for any disorder [40].

Willcutt and Pennington [43] sampled more than 200 twins who had RD and a matched sample with a mean age of 10.5 and found that subjects who had RD showed significantly elevated symptoms of ADHD, oppositional defiant disorder, conduct disorder, anxiety disorder, and mood disorder. After controlling for ADHD, none of the other disruptive behavior disorders were related significantly to RD; internalizing symptoms were not mediated by ADHD. There was a gender interaction, however: externalizing behaviors were related more strongly to boys who had RD and internalizing behaviors were related exclusively to girls who had RD. One consistent finding is that the inattentive type of ADHD is related more strongly to RD than either combined type or hyperactive/impulsive type [40,44].

There is considerable speculation about the nature of the relationship between disruptive behavior disorders and dyslexia. Several theories are forwarded, including unidirectional (reading problems cause behavioral disorders or vice versa) and bidirectional. Willcutt and coworkers [44] provide evidence for bivariate heritability between ADHD-I and RD, but not ADHD-Hyp/Imp. Trzesniewski and colleagues [42] also identify common genetic influences in ADHD-I and RD. Conversely, they report a reciprocal relationship between RD and antisocial behavior and the absence of heritability. In other words, reading problems contribute to acting-out behaviors, which in turn affect reading development negatively.

Although research into the relationship between disruptive behavior disorders and dyslexia is more prevalent and the link stronger, there is evidence that internalizing disorders also have a disproportionate impact on children who have dyslexia. Anxiety consistently is reported higher in subjects who have RD than in controls [40,43], with the greatest risk for generalized anxiety disorder and separation anxiety [40]. Data on mood disorders and RD are less consistent. Although clinically the general belief is that RD and depression are related, the data do not support this notion consistently. A reasonable conclusion from the data available is that boys who are dyslexic are at greater risk for showing externalizing symptoms broadly and girls are more likely to exhibit internalizing symptoms, especially anxiety. In view of the strong relationship between anxiety and mood disorders, however, the latter must be appreciated.

Assessing and diagnosing dyslexia

Although the assessment and diagnosis of learning disabilities (LD) at first glance may seem a straightforward process, the conceptualization of and guidelines for the identification of these disorders are evolving. Historically, LD has been defined as an unexpected problem learning in one or more of several academic areas and has been operationalized as a discrepancy between aptitude (as measured by IQ) and academic achievement. The *Diagnostic and Statistical Manual of Mental Disorders, Fourth Edition (DSM-IV)* [45] and the *International Classification of Diseases, Ninth Revision* [46] use a discrepancy definition for diagnosing learning disorders. As early as 1975, when Public Law 94-142 was implemented in the United States and LDs were considered a handicapping condition warranting special education services, the discrepancy model was one of the defining features. The same definition was adopted as part of the 1997 Individuals with Disabilities Education Act (IDEA). In the most recent IDEA revision, use of a discrepancy no longer is mandatory, although it is optional. Research to date is critical of this approach to defining and assessing any type of learning disorder. Discrepant (IQ > academic achievement scores) and nondiscrepant (nonmentally retarded but IQ not significantly discrepant from academic achievement) poor readers do not differ from each other in their response to educational interventions [47,48] or prognosis over time [49]. Empirically, there is no justification for using a discrepancy model for identifying a reading disorder. Many states and local education agencies continue to use this model for identifying and serving children as having LDs, however, and psychologists often continue to rely on the *DSM-IV* for guiding their assessment and diagnosis of LDs.

Intraindividual model

In view of the current state of practice and in an attempt to be proactive and forward looking, this article reviews the assessment process for reading disorders that is used most frequentlyand evidenced-based methods foreign to most pediatricians (although they will have to familiarize themselves with the process to understand individualized education plans [IEPs] they receive for their patients). Among elementary-aged children, assessment of reading skills requires, at minimum, objective measurement of word reading, reading fluency, and reading comprehension. Evaluation of word reading must include, in addition to reading whole words, reading of nonsense words that require application of phonics-based decoding skills (sounding words out). When evaluating children's ability to read words, they are presented simply with a list of words and asked to read them aloud. Similarly, assessing children's ability to use phonetic decoding requires patients to read a set of decodable nonsense words that that progressively are more difficult to read (eg, tib or blub). For younger children (eg, kindergarten and first grade), who are in the process of developing decoding skills, evaluation of skills critical to early reading is a better predictor of later reading problems than the actual measurement of word reading [27]. This includes evaluating phonologic awareness, working memory (memory span), serial naming, and expressive vocabulary. Each of these areas also should be covered in evaluations for children who are beyond the primary grades. Appreciating that reading the written word requires language and visual skills, assessment of orthographic coding is of value. Orthographic coding refers to children's ability to form mental images of words, letters, and letter strings [50], which in turn has an impact on their ability to recognize and retrieve the images rapidly. As outlined by Peterson and colleagues elsewhere in this issue, phonologic processing deficits are at the core of deficiency for the large majority of children who have dyslexia. Clinicians must be in a position to recognize deficits other than those considered typical reasons for a condition, however, because they may have a differential impact on recommended treatment.

Reading is a process that allows humans to access information and in turn increase knowledge. As such, the process of reading, to be most effective, should require minimal cognitive effort. Stated another way, eventually reading words should become a quick and automatic process. For children who are dyslexic, reading fluency often is the area most resistant to treatment and most persistant [51–53]. Many children who have RD develop adequate sight word reading vocabularies and even reasonable word decoding skills. The ability to read words quickly and efficiently, however, does not develop. Evaluating fluency is a critical component in any reading evaluation, especially beyond second grade.

Children's ability to understand what they read can result from several factors, including limited vocabulary [54], poor oral comprehension [55], and word reading deficits [28]. Not only must any reading disorder evaluation include a measure of reading comprehension, it is incumbent on evaluators to understand why children have poor comprehension skills. It is not sufficient to assume that children's reading comprehension problems are the result of decoding deficits exclusively if oral comprehension and vocabulary have not been measured. There is considerable evidence that children who have language impairment have not only comprehension deficits but also phonologic processing limitations that contribute to word reading deficits [56].

As discussed earlier, there is no empiric justification for using an IQ test to diagnose a learning disorder; however, that is not to say that a measure of cognitive functioning cannot contribute to a comprehensive evaluation.

Even if clinicians are comfortable that children's ability levels are within normal limits, there may be cognitive factors that help to explain reading difficulties. For example, most measures of intelligence include a vocabulary component, which plays a critical role in reading comprehension. Various memory dimensions also are included in IQ tests, again a factor that potentially could be helpful in diagnosing RDs and understanding why children are struggling to develop reading skills. Consequently, the constructive use of measures of cognitive functioning can contribute to a LD evaluation. Using an IQ test as a measure to identify the presence of absence of a discrepancy cannot be justified.

Response to intervention model

In the revision of the IDEA that took effect in 2005, the United States federal government included a Response to Intervention model as an empirically supported method to identifying LDs. Unlike the approach discussed previously, this model focuses on multiple short assessments to determine children's status and response to educational interventions. The idea behind this approach is that children at risk for reading problems (and learning problems in general) are identified early and provided with empirically supported treatments. Children are evaluated regularly to monitor progress and those not responding to interventions receive more intensive levels of service. Once it is determined that children have not responded to empirically supported methods of remediation, a diagnosis of a reading disorder is made. This article is not the venue for a comprehensive discussion of this model, yet it is important that pediatricians be aware of this approach, because many of their patients who have learning concerns may be involved in the process, which may be helpful to schools and possibly the children, but does not provide physicians with test results they are accustomed to reviewing (see Fletcher and colleagues [57] for a comprehensive review of assessment of LDs).

Pediatric evaluation and management of reading disability

It is not the responsibility of primary care physicians to make a diagnosis of dyslexia. Physicians often are the first to hear from parents worried about a child's academic progress. Furthermore, although referring children for an IEP team evaluation is a reasonable first step, teams at schools are in place not only to identify children's educational needs but also to determine if services should be provided. It is possible that children may have a LD, such as dyslexia, but do not qualify for any type of service. There also is a range of services that may be available within a specific school system. For example, all schools have early intervention programs for reading and most for math. Involvement with a reading specialist at this level may be the best option for children at that time. The issue not necessarily where the child receives reading assistance (special education versus a reading specialist) but the type of intervention provided.

Being aware of a family history of language or reading problems is critical. Children who have positive family histories or who show other early risk factors should be considered for evaluation or for an interventional plan. Finding out from parents if their 4- or 5- year-old child is reciting nursery rhymes or interested in playing rhyming games provides an approximate indication of early phonemic sensitivity. Pediatricians even can ask 5-year-old children to produce a few rhyming words (eg, "Tell me a real word that rhymes with ball...mat...car," and so forth). By the end of kindergarten, are children able to recognize lower and upper case letters of the alphabet and are they beginning to associate sounds with letters? Again, in addition to asking parents, physicians can screen by showing children randomly a few letters and asking them to name them and identify the associated sounds. Asking parents if their first-grade child is beginning to apply phonetic decoding skills gives an idea if the child has begun to apply what should be being taught at school. Avoidance or lack of interest in reading, especially when paired with observed (either by parents or teachers) reading difficulties should be cause for concern. It is better to intervene early; evidence to date suggests that taking a wait-and-see approach to reading seldom is successful [19,49,52].

Interested pediatricians have access to screening measures for learning difficulties [58]. One such resource is the Wide Range Achievement Test 4 (WRAT4) [59]. This instrument has solid psychometric properties and includes a nationally represented normative sample for individuals ages 5 through adulthood. The WRAT4 consists of three subtests that measure word reading, spelling, and arithmetic calculations. Administration time is approximately 10 to 15 minutes. Adequate performance on either the word reading or the spelling component does not rule out dyslexia. Poor performance, however (ie, below a standard score of 90), in the context of reading concerns reported by teachers or parents may warrant a referral for a comprehensive evaluation by a psychologist or neuropsychologist. The two cases in this article present common patient concerns expressed to pediatricians.

Summary

Reading skills progress in a stage-like manner, like many other developmental processes. There is no evidence that reading, unlike language, develops without direct instruction. Failing to develop preceding skills has a dramatic impact on development of more sophisticated reading skills. For example, children who have poor phonemic sensitivity struggle to develop phonetic decoding; poor word recognition and word decoding skills have a negative impact on reading comprehension. Primary care physicians need to be aware of reading and potential reading problems and frequent comorbid conditions. Awareness and recognition of risk factors can help physicians direct children early to badly needed resources. Although there is no guarantee that remediation of reading problems allows children to avoid co-occurring and comorbid conditions often associated with dyslexia, at the least it decreases the risk for and minimizes the impact of one additional challenge for these children.

Case 1

History and symptom presentation

Jim is a 9-year-old African American boy who just began third grade. Parents and teachers always have believed he was making adequate academic progress in all areas. In fact, parents stated that he was "reading" books at 5 years of age, and although he struggled somewhat with second grade–level books, he was able to understand the material well. They gave examples of him laughing while lying in bed and reading a few of the books in the *Captain Underpants* series. When asked what was so funny, he was able to tell his parents all about the story and the potty humor that was so appealing. Third grade has been a challenge, however. His third grade teacher had been told by previous teachers that Jim was bright and needed to be challenged, yet the teacher was perplexed because Jim did not like to read aloud during reading group and began to act silly and goofy during those times. When evaluating his reading skills informally, the third grade teacher placed Jim in the lowest reading group, explaining to his parents that he had good "strategies" for reading words, including use of picture cues and context cues to figure out words; however, he seldom applied phonetic decoding principals.

Test results

Jim's pediatrician referred him for a private psychologic evaluation. On interview, it was determined that although there was no family history of reading or language deficits, Jim's father had never read a novel in his life. He reads the newspaper but finds that reading takes too long and tends to get most news from the local TV station or CNBC. His father also indicated that he relies heavily on spell check when sending email messages at work. Jim's mother said that when she and her husband first were married she could not decipher his spelling, although over the years she has gotten pretty good at doing so. Testing with Jim indicated strong language skills, including oral comprehension and vocabulary skills that were in the 80th percentile. When reading aloud, he could not read the word "erupt," and therefore could not answer the comprehension question correctly. Later, when asked what the word "erupt" meant, he defined the word easily. Reading of whole words fell in the 16th percentile, which is considered low average, but reading of nonsense words, words that require phonetic decoding, fell in the second percentile. Not surprisingly, phonemic awareness skills fell in the fifth percentile. Test results support the hypothesis that as a youngster Jim was memorizing books and relying on whole words he was able to memorize. When the reading demands increased, he was unable to keep pace with same-grade peers, despite his strong language skills.

Disposition

Jim was diagnosed with dyslexia and qualified for special education services for children who have a specific RD. No comorbid conditions were identified. He began receiving special education services, but because a comprehensive and systematic approach to word reading was not being applied, even after multiple attempts on the part of the parents and the clinician to encourage the LD teacher to do so, the decision was made to seek outside reading assistance from a dyslexia specialist. Although this added an hour to Jim's school day 3 times a week, because he recognized gains and liked the tutor, he generally was okay with attending.

Case 2

History and symptom presentation

Shelly was a delightful, energetic 6-year-old white girl. She was midway through first grade when her parents received a call from the teacher expressing concerns about Shelly's behavior in the classroom. The teacher noticed that Shelly did not seem to understand and follow directions. He gave examples of the class transitioning from spelling to math and Shelly having her spelling material out when the other kids had their math books on their desk. When she looked at the kids in the seats next to her and saw that their math books were out, she quickly would pull out the correct book. The teacher also noticed that Shelly's verbal responses to questions tended to be brief and include minimal verbiage. Although she was developing some sight words when reading, the teacher noted that Shelly still did not recognize a few lower case letters consistently and also continued to mix up the upper case letters, B and D, when asked to identify them orally. The teacher estimated that Shelly was able to identify approximately 65% of letters' sounds.

Test results

The school initiated an IEP team evaluation. The school psychologist found that Shelly's IQ was in the low-average range, reporting the following scores from the Wechsler Intelligence Scale for Children—Fourth Edition [60]: full scale IQ 89, verbal comprehension index 79, perceptual reasoning index 110, working memory index 86, and processing speed index 91. The LD diagnostician administered the Woodcock-Johnson III Tests of Achievement (WJ-III) [61]. All reading measure scores were in the low to mid 80s, where the mean is 100 with a SD of 15. The sound awareness subtest from the WJ-III also was administered, which evaluates different types of phonemic awareness; Shelly earned a standard score of 79. The school reasoned that Shelly's reading scores were commensurate with cognitive functioning and, therefore, she did not have a LD.

Shelly then was seen privately because the parents believed they were getting little direction from the school. On review of the testing completed through the school, it was determined that little additional cognitive or educational testing was needed; rather, Shelly was referred for a language evaluation. The speech/language pathologist reported scores of receptive language that fell in the 14th percentile and expressive language in the third percentile. Additional evaluation of phonologic processing identified, as expected, severely deficient phonemic awareness and phonologic memory. Test results were presented to the school and an alternative interpretation of the original evaluation was suggested; that is, her low overall cognitive functioning was a reflection of language deficits and related memory concerns, not intelligence.

Disposition

The school agreed with the alternative interpretation of the original test results and accepted the language evaluation completed through the hospital. Shelly was diagnosed with a mixed receptive-expressive language disorder and began language therapy through school twice a week. School personnel still did not believe that she met the criteria of children who have a LD but agreed that Shelly needed early intervention services, and she began working with a reading specialist 3 times a week. The speech/language pathologist and reading specialist consult with each other to coordinate services to make sure phonologic processing skills are addressed and match up with instruction in sound/symbol correspondence.

References

[1] Snow C, Adams M, Bowman B, et al. Preventing reading difficulties in young children. Washington, DC: National Academy Press; 1998.
[2] Lyon GR, Fletcher JM, Barnes M. Learning disabilities. In: Marsh EJ, Barkley RA, editors. Child psychopathology. 2nd edition. New York: Guilford Press; 2002. p. 520–88.
[3] Adams MJ. Beginning to read: thinking and learning about pring. Cambridge (MA): MIT Press; 1990.
[4] National Reading Panel. Teaching children to read: an evidence-based assessment of the scientific research literature on reading and its implications for reading instruction. Jessup (MD): EDPubs; 2000.
[5] Snow CE, Barnes W, Chandler J, et al. Unfulfilled expectations: home and school influences on literacy. Cambridge (MA): Harvard; 1991.
[6] Vellutino FR, Scanlon DM, Tanzman MS. Bridging the gap between cognitive and neuropsychological conceptualizations of reading disability. Learn Individ Differ 1991;3:181–203.
[7] Wagner RK, Torgeson JK, Rashotte CA, et al. Changing causal relations between phonological processing abilities and word-level reading as children develop from beginning to skilled readers: a 5-year longitudinal study. Child Dev 1997;33:468–79.
[8] Lonigan CJ, Burgess SR, Anthony JL. Development of emergent literacy and early reading skills in preschool children: evidence from a latent-variable longitudinal study. Dev Psychol 2000;36:596–613.
[9] Foorman B, Anthony J, Seals L, et al. Language development and emergent literacy in preschool. Semin Pediatr Neurol 2002;9:173–84.
[10] Stevenson HW, Newman RS. Long-term prediction of achievement and attitudes in mathematics and reading. Child Dev 1986;57:646–59.
[11] Burgess SR, Lonigan CJ. Bidirectional relations of phonologicl sensitivity and prereading skills: evidence from a preschool sample. J Exp Child Psychol 1998;70:117–41.
[12] Snowling MJ. Dyslexia. Oxford (UK): Blackwell; 2000.

[13] Byrnes J. Minds, brains, and learning: understanding the psychological and educational relevance of neuroscientific research. New York: Guilford Press; 2001.

[14] Tabors PO, Roach KA, Snow CE. Home language and literacy environment: final results. In: Dickinson DK, Tabors PO, editors. Beginning literacy with language: young children learning at home and school. Baltimore (MD): Paul H. Brooes Publishing; 2001. p. 111–38.

[15] Hess RD, Holloway S. Family and school as educational institutions. In: Parke RD, editor. Review of child development research, 7: the family. Chicago: University of Chicago Press; 1984. p. 179–222.

[16] Schatschneider C, Torgeson JK. Using our current understanding of dyslexia to support early identification and intervention. J Child Neurol 2004;19:759–65.

[17] Scanlon DM, Vellutino FR. Prerequisite skills, early instruction, and success in first grade reading: selected results from a longitudinal study. Ment Retard Dev Disabil Res Rev 1996;2:54–63.

[18] Stanovich KE. Matthew effects in reading: some consequences of individual differences in the acquisition of literacy. Reading Research Quarterly 1986;21:360–407.

[19] Juel C. Learning to read and write: a longitudinal study of 54 children from first through fourth grades. J Educ Psychol 1988;80:434–47.

[20] Chall JS, Jacobs V, Baldwin L. The reading crisis: why poor children fall behind. Cambridge (MA): Harvard University Press; 1990.

[21] Kaplan DS, Liu X, Kaplan HB. Influence of parents' self-feelings and expectations on children's academic performance. J Educ Res 2001;94:360–70.

[22] Stanovich KE, Cunningham AE, Feeman DJ. Intelligence, cognitive skills and early reading progress. Reading Research Quarterly 1984;19:278–303.

[23] Juel C. Beginning reading. In: Barr R, Kamil ML, Mosenthal PB, et al, editors. Handbook of reading research, vol. 2. Mahwah (NJ): Lawrence Earlbaum Associates; 1991. p. 759–88.

[24] Wagner RK, Torgeson JK, Rashotte CA. Development of reading-related phonological processing abilities: new evidence of bidirectional causality from a latent variable longitudinal study. Dev Psychol 1994;30:73–87.

[25] Bishop DV, Adams C. A prospective study of the relationship between specific language impairment, phonological disorders and reading retardation. J Child Psychol Psychiatry 1990; 31:1027–50.

[26] Snowling MJ, Bishop DV, Stothard SE. Is preschool language impairment a risk factor for dyslexia in adolescence? J Child Psychol Psychiatry 2000;41:587–600.

[27] Scarborough H. Connecting early language and literacy to later reading (dis)abilities: evidence, theory and practice. In: Neuman SB, Dickinson DK, editors. Handbook of early literacy research. New York: Guilford Press; 2001. p. 97–110.

[28] Stanovich KE. Progress in understanding reading: scientific foundations and new frontiers. New York: Guilford Press; 2000.

[29] Schmidt HP, Kuryliw AJ, Saklofske DH, et al. Stability of WISC–R scores for a sample of learning disabled children. Psychol Rep 1989;64:195–201.

[30] Fawcett AJ. Dyslexia, the cerebellum and phonological skill. In: Witruk E, Friederici AD, Lachmann T, editors. Basic functions of language, reading and reading disability. Dordrecht (Netherlands): Kluwer Academic Publishers; 2002. p. 265–79.

[31] Fawcett AJ, Nicolson RI, Maclagan F. Cerebellar tests differentiate between groups of poor readers with and without IQ discrepancy. J Learn Disabil 2001;34:119–35.

[32] Kooistra L, Crawford S, Dewey D, et al. Motor correlates of ADHD: contribution of reading disability and oppositional defiant disorder. J Learn Disabil 2005;38:195–206.

[33] Iversen S, Berg K, Ellertsen B, et al. Motor coordination difficulties in a municipality group and in a clinical sample of poor readers. Dyslexia: An International Journal of Research and Practice 2005;11:217–31.

[34] Bruininks RH. Bruininks-Oseretsky test of motor proficiency. Circle Pines (MN): American Guidance Service; 1978.

[35] Beery KE. The developmental test of visual-motor integration. 3rd edition. Cleveland (OH): Modern Curriculum Press; 1989.

[36] Berninger VW, Fuller F, Whitaker D. A process model of writing development across the life span. Educational Psychology Review 1997;8:193–238.

[37] Berninger VW, Yates C, Cartwright A, et al. Lower-level developmental skills in beginning writing. Reading and Writing: An Interdisciplinary Journal 1992;4:257–80.

[38] Berninger VW. Understanding the "graphia" in developmental dysgraphia: a developmental neuropsychological perspective for disorders in producing written language. In: Dewey D, Tupper DE, editors. Developmental motor disorders: a neuropsychological perspective. New York: Guilford Press; 2004. p. 328–50.

[39] Berninger VW, Amtmann KR. Preventing written expression disabilities through early and continuing assessment and intervention for handwriting and/or spelling problems: research into practice. In: Swanson HL, Harris KR, Graham S, editors. Handbook of learning disabilities. New York: Guilford Press; 2003. p. 345–63.

[40] Carroll JM, Maughan B, Goodman R, et al. Literacy difficulties and psychiatric disorders: evidence for comorbidity. J Child Psychol Psychiatry 2005;46:524–32.

[41] Hinshaw SP. Externalizing behavior problems and academic underachievement in childhood and adolescence: causal relationships and underlying mechanisms. Psychol Bull 1992;111:127–55.

[42] Trzesniewski KH, Moffitt TE, Caspi A, et al. Revisiting the association between reading achievement and antisocial behavior: new evidence of an environmental explanation from a twin study. Child Dev 2006;77:72–88.

[43] Willcutt EG, Pennington BF. Psychiatric comorbidity in children and adolescents with reading disability. J Child Psychol Psychiatry 2000;41:1039–48.

[44] Willcutt EG, Pennington BF, DeFries JC. Twin study of the etiology of comorbidity between reading disability and attention-deficit/hyperactivity disorder. Am J Med Genet B Neuropsychiatr Genet 2000;96:293–301.

[45] American Psychiatric Association. Diagnostic and statistical manual of mental disorders. 4th edition. Washington, DC: American Psychiatric Association; 1994.

[46] World Health Organization. International classification of diseases. 9th edition. World Health Organization; 2004.

[47] Fletcher JM, Lyon GR, Barnes M, et al. Classification of learning disabilities: an evidence-based approach. In: Bradley R, Danielson L, Hallahan DP, editors. Identification of learning disabilities: research to practice. Mahway (NJ): Lawrence Erlbaum Associates; 2002. p. 185–250.

[48] Stage SA, Abbott RD, Jenkins JR, et al. Predicting response to early reading intervention from verbal IQ, reading-related language abilities, attention ratings, and verbal IQ-word readings discrepancy: failure to validate discrepancy method. J Learn Disabil 2003;36:24–33.

[49] Francis DJ, Shaywitz SE, Stuebing KK, et al. Developmental lag versus deficit models of reading disability: a longitudinal, individual growth curves analysis. J Educ Psychol 1996;88:3–17.

[50] Mather N, Goldstein S. Learning disabilities and challenging behaviors: a guide to intervention and classroom management. Baltimore (MD): Paul H. Brookes; 2001.

[51] Shaywitz SE, Fletcher JM, Holahan JM, et al. Persistence of dyslexia: the Connecticut longitudinal study at adolescence. Pediatrics 1999;104:1351–9.

[52] Torgeson JK, Alexander AW, Wagner RK, et al. Intensive remedial instruction for children with severe reading disabilities: immediate and long-term outcomes from two instructional approaches. J Learn Disabil 2001;34:33–58.

[53] Wolf M, Bowers PG. Naming speed processes, timing and reading: a conceptual review. J Learn Disabil 1999;33:387–407.

[54] Hirsch ED. Reading comprehension requires knowledge—of words and the world. American Educator 2003;10–31.

[55] Biemiller A. Oral comprehension sets the ceiling on reading comprehension. American Educator 2003;1–3.

[56] Catts HW, Fey ME, Tomblin JB, et al. A longitudinal investigation of reading outcomes in children with language impairments. J Speech Lang Hear Res 2002;45:1142–57.

[57] Fletcher JM, Francis DJ, Morris RD, et al. Evidenced-based assessment of learning disabilities in children and adolescents. J Clin Child Adolesc Psychol 2005;34:506–22.

[58] Grizzle KL, Simms MD. Early language development and language learning disabilities. Pediatr Rev 2005;26:274–83.

[59] Wilkinson GS, Robertson GJ. Wide range achievement test. 4th edition. East Aurora (NY): Slosson; 2006.

[60] Wechsler D. Wechsler intelligence scale for children. 4th edition. San Antonio (TX): The Psychological Corporation; 2003.

[61] Woodcock RW, McGrew KS, Mather N. Woodcock-Johnson III tests of achievement. 3rd edition. Riverside (CA): Riverside Publishing; 2001.

ELSEVIER
SAUNDERS

PEDIATRIC CLINICS
OF NORTH AMERICA

Pediatr Clin N Am 54 (2007) 525–542

Language Impairment and Psychiatric Comorbidities

Nancie Im-Bolter, PhD[a],*, Nancy J. Cohen, PhD[b]

[a]Department of Psychology, Otonabee College, Trent University,
Peterborough, Ontario, Canada K9J 7B8
[b]Hincks-Dellcrest Institute, Department of Psychiatry, University of Toronto,
114 Maitland Street, Toronto, ON M4Y 1E1, Canada

Children develop the capacity to understand and use language in a relatively short time. This development has a significant impact on children's thinking, learning, and social relationships. Language helps children organize their perceptions, sharpen their memories, and learn about their world. Social development also is facilitated by language once children are able to communicate wishes, views, and intentions. Even earlier, children's ability to communicate with gestures is a precursor to language and social interaction. Language also provides a personal function by helping children express their emotions, organize their behavior, and understand their experiences. When language does not develop normally, quality of life across the age span is affected and many children who have language impairment (LI) suffer long-term consequences in their academic, social, and emotional well-being [1]. Approximately 50% of children seen in mental health clinics and in special classrooms for children who have social-emotional problems have LI, with estimates as high as 70% [2]. Similarly, on average, half of the children referred to speech-language pathologists or to special education classes for learning disabilities have a social-emotional problem [3]. Although there is an increased awareness of the relationship between LI and social-emotional disorders, researchers and clinicians continue to struggle with distinguishing between language-related and -nonrelated behaviors. It is important to understand how one might be confused, or interact, with the other to optimize identification, assessment, and treatment in clinical practice.

This article first provides an overview of LI and its associated conditions and proceeds to discuss the interactive relationship between language and

---

* Corresponding author.
E-mail address: nimbolter@trentu.ca (N. Im-Bolter).

other domains of development. The way in which LI has an impact on adjustment depends on the developmental tasks children are struggling with at a particular point in time. Consequently, the framework of developmental psychopathology is used to organize this discussion. This framework emphasizes that there are transactions between developmental domains within individuals and their environment. This article focuses on children who have LI who do not have a diagnosis of general developmental delay or who do not have significant structural brain injury, autism, or developmental disorder. Throughout, how knowledge can be translated to practice is highlighted.

Overview of terminology and associated conditions

Language impairment

Currently, the terms LI or specific language impairment, are used most commonly to refer to problems in the acquisition and use of language in the context of normal development not associated with any other clinical condition [4]. Because this criterion is debated and research indicates that children who have LI have impairments in the cognitive domain even when little or no language is involved [5,6], the term LI is used in this article.

Preverbal communication

Even before oral language develops, infants achieve certain cognitive milestones that prepare them for language. For example, preverbal infants learn to think about means and ends (intentional behaviors that achieve a goal, such as pulling on a cloth to retrieve a toy) and show a capacity for deferred imitation (copying an action after a delay), which requires the construction, storage, and retrieval of mental symbols. These cognitive achievements reflect symbolic thought and help prepare infants to use words as symbolic tools of communication [6]. Observations of infant play can help determine if means and ends and deferred imitation behaviors are in place.

The ability to communicate for social purposes is a crucial part of development from birth onward. In infancy, the overlap between communicative and social-emotional development is most evident. For example, important developmental achievements that occur between 9 and 12 months of age are joint attention and shared reference. These behaviors refer to infants' use of communicative means (such as smiles or gestures) intentionally to gain and guide attention of others toward objects and events. Gestures, pointing, and gaze direction are precursors to language development; infants use them to make themselves understood and become involved in social interactions. They also begin to understand when they must repair a failed communication, that is, try another strategy to gain the attention of others when one strategy does not work. Infants who have little or no appreciable use of gestures (such as pointing) at 18 months should be referred for formal developmental assessment that includes a hearing test.

Early social interactions depend on competent infant behavior and sensitive, responsive caregivers. If infants do not respond to or initiate joint attention interactions, this may disturb the infant-caregiver relationship. Joint attention is associated with infants' capacity to initiate shared positive affective states with significant others. As a result, problems with joint attention may foreshadow social-emotional and language difficulties. Observations of play interactions between infants and caregivers can be helpful in determining whether or not difficulties with joint attention or shared reference exist. Questionnaires and checklists also can be used with parents to obtain information on their infants' gestural expression and understanding (eg, MacArthur-Bates Communicative Development Inventories [7] and Communication and Symbolic Behavior Scales [8]). When observations suggest social-emotional concerns, referral to an infant mental health specialist and a developmental/language specialist should be considered.

Verbal communication

Infants typically say their first word near their first birthday and this marks a major turning point in their ability to communicate, learn, engage in social interactions, and regulate their emotions and behavior. As infants begin to talk, there is more complexity in terms of what needs to be attended to, with respect to language and associated developmental capacities.

The larger system of language includes speech, which refers to the physical production of the sounds of a language. Problems, such as inaccurate articulation, stuttering, stammering, and unusual voice, are examples of speech impairments. These problems are distinct from language problems and only in a minority of cases do developmental speech impairments reflect LI [9]. Consequently, speech impairments are not discussed.

Language has two main modalities, receptive (comprehension or understanding) and expressive (production), each divided into three structural components: phonology (sound system of language), semantics (meaning of words and word combinations), and grammar (rules for the combination of words and sentences). Another aspect of receptive language, auditory verbal processing, also typically is considered. Although language can be described in this fine-grained way, children learn all these components of language simultaneously. Also, in daily language use, they are intimately interrelated.

Children who have LI often have problems with receptive and expressive language. In terms of development, by 1 year of age, children are able to recognize and discriminate the sounds of their native language (phonology). Children who have LI are found to demonstrate deficits in awareness of the speech sounds of language (phonological awareness). Phonological awareness is shown to predict later problems in reading [10]. Even earlier, in the preschool years, problems in phonological awareness can be discerned in children who have difficulty understanding and creating rhymes.

By their first birthday, children not only understand words but also begin to use words to communicate (semantics or vocabulary). A good vocabulary facilitates literacy skills and social communication. By 3 years of age, normally developing children have an expressive vocabulary of approximately 1000 words and a receptive vocabulary of close to 50,000 words. Children who have LI often are late in saying their first words and, thus, have difficulty expressing themselves. In time, they typically master the direct, concrete, and simple meanings of words but have difficulty with the indirect, abstract, and complex meanings of words. When children's vocabulary is limited, their ability to express themselves and to understand others also is limited. As a result, children can be perceived by teachers, clinicians, other adults, and even children as resistant, shy, withdrawn, refusing to speak, or reluctant to answer. As a result, misattributions can occur when children who have these behaviors are not meeting expectations in school. It is important to rule out language difficulties and associated cognitive problems, even though, superficially, underachievement may not seem to be learning based. Research shows that treatment can improve children's language skills, but early intervention is critical [9].

The grammatical aspect of language is represented by the rules of word order and combinations and the use of correct word endings and forms to indicate verb tense. Children who have LI tend to use shorter sentences and have difficulties understanding and producing grammatically complex sentences with elaborated verb phrases, pronouns, adjectives, and auxiliaries [4]. Thus, most children do not have difficulty understanding the simple sentence, "The boy saw the cat," but may encounter more difficulty with sentences that have embedded phrases and passive verb tense, for instance, "The cat sleeping under the chair was seen by the boy." These sorts of deficits can have an impact on overall communicative competence by impeding the ability to derive meaning from text and social interactions. This necessarily interferes with social relationships, education, and therapy.

Auditory verbal processing, or the ability to analyze verbal input, also is important for competent language performance. Children who have LI have well documented deficits in processing verbal information efficiently [11]. These problems manifest in slowed or inaccurate information processing. In classrooms, children who have LI may understand only one request at a time, have trouble remembering steps in problem-solving tasks, or miss some of the instructions for homework. As a result, it is understandable that children begin to "tune out" or seem to have attention problems. Problems with verbal processing can be exacerbated if verbal information is loaded emotionally, is complex syntactically, contains unfamiliar vocabulary, or must be decoded and interpreted quickly, as is the case in classrooms, in many social interactions, and in therapy. For instance, when children fail to carry out a series of directions completely, it sometimes is attributed by adults as noncompliance or "doing only what they want to do." This can have a profound effect on children's self-confidence and self-esteem. It is important in this context to note that a hearing screening should be a routine part of language assessments. Children who seem to be not listening actually might be not hearing.

The use of language for learning and communication goes beyond the level of individual words or sentences. Three integrative aspects of language increasingly become important as children mature—pragmatics, narrative discourse, and higher-order language. Pragmatic skills are observed when individuals engage in social interactions, the connected and contingent flow of language between two or more individuals. The ability to initiate and sustain social interaction requires the integration of verbal and nonverbal pragmatic skills with structural language and with social-cognitive and cognitive skills. Verbal pragmatic skills include the ability to (1) initiate conversation, (2) take turns, (3) maintain a topic, (4) shift to different topics when required, (5) request conversational repair (ie, ask for further information or clarification), (6) respond to conversational repair requests, (7) produce language that is appropriate to context and situation, and (8) narrate experiences and events. Nonverbal pragmatic skills include facial expression, gestures, eye contact, and physical proximity to a conversational partner. Children who have LI have difficulties with verbal and nonverbal pragmatic skills, which can cause increasing difficulties with peers and have an impact on their ability to form friendships. Narrative discourse skills are an important part of social interactions, as children need to be able to relate personal experiences, stories, and events in a logically consistent and sequential manner. The narratives of children who have LI tend to refer to people, objects, or events in an ambiguous or unclear manner, are sequenced inappropriately, and tend to be short and descriptive rather than explanatory and goal oriented [12]. Nonverbal pragmatic skills refer to the physical, emotional, and gestural aspects of communication that complement, expand, reinforce, or even contradict what is said verbally.

Finally, higher-order (figurative) language increasingly becomes essential as children move into adolescence and need to become competent in understanding and using nonliteral forms of language (eg, "Cut that out"). Other aspects of figurative language include understanding metaphors, sarcasm, teasing, and jokes and the ability to discuss abstract topics, such as politics or art. This form of language is thought to be critically important to adolescent academic and social life. Success in school is found to be associated with students' skills with figurative language [13]. Also, the ability to use slang and jargon (based primarily on figurative language) is associated with peer acceptance and the ability to establish friendships [13]. Little research has been done on the figurative language skills of children who have LI and none on adolescents who have LI [14].

Language and other domains of development

In the normal course of development, language is intertwined with abilities in the cognitive, social, and emotional domains (and vice versa). These domains do not develop simply in parallel but influence each other on an ongoing basis so that, for example, developments in language may affect understanding of emotion, which in turn influences social interactional skills. Competence in one area, therefore, may be necessary for the emergence of capacities in another [15]. Normal development can be construed as the integration of earlier competences into a later stage of development and atypical development as the lack of integration of the different areas due to deficits or difficulties [16]. Although the focus is on language, competence in each domain contributes to competence in the others. There are critical cognitive, social-cognitive, and emotional tasks associated with language across development. Most relevant to this discussion of LI and psychopathology are social cognition and emotional development. In terms of practice, assessment should encompass this range of functioning, and practitioners and educators need to be aware of the interrelated conditions.

Social cognition

Social cognition is a broad term that refers to the cognitive processes individuals apply in social situations and includes social problem solving. In order to solve social problems and maintain harmonious relations with peers, children must be able to reflect on and talk about feelings, be able to understand that there might be many ways to see a situation, realize how their intentions might be viewed by others, and appreciate that coordinating different perspectives and responding to social expectations and cues are important for successful peer relationships. Competent social problem solving requires the successful integration of various skills in the cognitive, emotional, and language domains. Few studies have examined social problem solving in children who have LI, but the handful that exist suggest that children who have LI have problems negotiating with others and resolving conflicts [17].

A review of longitudinal research indicates that immaturity in social problem solving may play a role in the development of psychopathology [18]. A recent study indicates that language plays a mediating role between social problem solving and psychopathology [18]. This suggests that over time, language deficits could affect the development of social problem-solving skills adversely, leading to an increased risk for psychopathology. Most social-cognitive interventions are language based, and the language skills of children referred to such programs rarely are assessed.

Emotional development

Language is not only a tool for thought and social interaction but also a means to control one's own behavior and emotions and those of others. More specifically, language plays a role in enabling children to understand, encode, organize, and retrieve rules that contribute to emotional and behavioral regulation. From a developmental perspective, it is not surprising that parents seek help with managing and understanding behavior problems when there is a clash between children's developmental needs and parental expectations. Children who are able to say, "I am mad" or "I am sad," are more likely to gain the support and understanding of adults than those who throw temper tantrums or hit other children. As language develops, children begin to discuss their emotions with their caregivers and, in turn, their caregivers help them deal constructively with negative emotions by talking about them. These supportive conversations facilitate children's capacity to devise their own strategies to regulate their emotions.

Self-directed talk, which appears at approximately 2 years, provides a means for coping with unpleasant emotions by turning attention away from frightening events ("Scary cave, don't want to see it!"), by replacing unpleasant thoughts with pleasant ones ("Mommy's gone, but she'll be back soon"), by helping to reinterpret causes of distress ("That witch is mean, but she's just pretending right?"), by controlling and modulating arousal to accomplish a goal ("Slowly, slowly"), and by facilitating the expression of emotional states ("Broke glass, mommy angry?"). Later, self-directed talk also can provide a tool for reflection, description, and self-questioning that contributes to cognitive and social-cognitive problem solving [19]. Disruptions in language development are likely to have a negative impact on the development of self-directed talk and, therefore, the ability to use self-directed talk in a variety of emotionally laden situations.

Children who have good emotion regulation are more likely to be good problem solvers, compromise, and meet mutual needs when playing with peers; to be able to make new friends; and to develop social interaction skills in play. In contrast, children who do not learn how to regulate emotions are likely to alienate adults and peers when they act out their anger or frustrations physically rather than use their language to communicate in a more appropriate way.

Language impairment: the invisible handicap

LI has been called a "marginal" or "invisible" handicap because often it is subtle and cannot be determined without a thorough assessment. In addition, children who have LI can seem to demonstrate contradictory language abilities (eg, having knowledge but showing inconsistent performance) and show day-to-day variability in their ability to communicate. In informal conversational settings, children can use one-word responses and grammatically simple or well-learned sentences and be understood. Furthermore, informal use of language usually entails speaking on topics of one's own choice. This helps explain why much of what children who have LI say spontaneously can be correct grammatically [20].

When language expression or comprehension is required "on demand," as is the case in school, children are required to coordinate linguistic, cognitive, social, and emotional information. More specifically, children who do not answer when asked a question or seem distracted in a classroom may seem, to adults, to be noncompliant, inattentive, or socially withdrawn. These latter symptoms actually may be related to problems with producing or understanding language. Because LI can be subtle, children may be diagnosed inaccurately, for instance with oppositional and conduct disorders, without any assessment of their language skills. It is critical in these instances that children's language and cognitive skills are assessed to understand how these abilities may be affecting or interacting with observed behaviors.

Prevalence of language impairment

It is estimated that 8% to 12% of preschool children have some form of LI [21] and that the prevalence of LI in kindergarten children ranges from 8% to 13% [22,23]. There are fewer data on the prevalence of LI in older children and adolescents. In the age range of 6 to 21 years, the prevalence rates typically are 5%, although figures as high as 20% are cited [9]. Even when less stringent diagnostic criteria are used, however, associations between LI and concurrent and later learning and social-emotional problems are reported [24,25]. Children who have LI often are referred initially for assessment and treatment because they are "late talkers." Many children who exhibit mild and early language problems seem to catch up to their peers; however, research shows that, in some, residual effects of early LI may be evident in later childhood and adolescence, at times when demands on language for tasks such as inferential reading skills and understanding and using nonliteral language are required. Tests of language available for older children often do not adequately assess or measure the complex and abstract language skills necessary to perform well in middle childhood and beyond. As a result, it is likely that the residual effects of LI in older children are greater than reported. Children who have LI should have regular reassessments and follow-up, even when their LI seems resolved, to ensure the detection of problems as language demands (and the language environment) change with age.

Psychiatric disorders and language impairment

The classification system used most widely for psychiatric disorders in North America is the American Psychiatric Association's *Diagnostic and Statistical Manual of Mental Disorders, Revised Fourth Edition* (*DSM-IV-R*) [26]. This article uses the terminology used in the *DSM-IV-R* for ease of discussion, although children who do not meet criteria for a psychiatric (or social-emotional) disorder still can be impaired in their social-emotional functioning. Language plays a central role in child psychiatric populations, as most therapies are verbally based, including the cognitive behavioral and social skills training techniques often applied to children who have attention-deficit/hyperactivity disorder (ADHD). Language skills rarely are evaluated systematically before such therapies are undertaken, so caution should be exercised in attributing to children who have psychiatric disorders what might be a reflection of problems for children who have LI [27].

LI commonly is associated with ADHD, conduct disorder, oppositional defiant disorder, anxiety disorder, depression, and anxiety [9]. As these psychiatric disorders are discussed in more detail, it becomes evident that many of the symptoms that characterize psychiatric disorders just as well could be considered indicative of LI.

Attention-deficit/hyperactivity disorder

The most common psychiatric diagnosis observed in children who have LI is ADHD. In the authors' research, for instance, in 7- to 14-year-old children presenting as child psychiatric outpatients and who met criteria for LI, 46% had a diagnosis of ADHD [28]. This diagnosis is characterized by problems with inattention, hyperactivity, and impulsivity that impair social or academic functioning. When looking at the specific psychiatric symptoms for ADHD, there is potential overlap with pragmatic language and language processing. For example, symptoms of inattention include "does not seem to listen when spoken to" and "does not follow through on instructions or duties"; symptoms of hyperactivity include "talks incessantly"; and symptoms of impulsivity include "blurts outs answers before questions have been completed" and "interrupts others." The authors' research shows that verbal and nonverbal working memory deficits are associated more closely with LI than ADHD [27] and that deficits in inhibitory control (hypothesized to be a core deficit in children who have ADHD) are found in children who have LI [5].

Disruptive behavior disorders: oppositional defiant disorder and conduct disorder

The diagnoses of oppositional defiant disorder and conduct disorder are applied to children who exhibit oppositional and disruptive behavior. Conduct disorder is more serious and appears later in development. It often includes aggressive and delinquent behavior.

Oppositional defiant disorder is described as a pattern of negative, hostile, and defiant behavior that is more frequent than expected of children of comparable age and developmental level. It often is accompanied by such pragmatic language deficits as poor topic maintenance, poor negotiation skills, and inadequate interpretation of verbal and nonverbal social communication [29]. Clinically and empirically, it is known that adults can overestimate toddlers' language ability and may attribute problems with language comprehension to willful disobedience. In fact, toddlers' compliance with adults' commands is related directly to toddlers' receptive language ability [30]. It is likely that the relationship between compliance to commands and receptive language ability exists in older children.

To be diagnosed with conduct disorder, children must demonstrate a repetitive, persistent pattern of behavior that violates the basic rights of others (eg, destruction of property, serious violation of rules, or theft). Conduct disorder, including delinquency, is associated with LI [31], including pragmatic LI [32]. Early and ongoing problems have detrimental effects on children's behavior (eg, increasing frustration at not being understood or able to affect other's behaviors or difficulty using language for self-regulation), relationship with caregivers, ability to benefit from learning in school, and relationships with peers.

Mood and anxiety disorders

Depression can interfere with communication, memory, and auditory processing. It also can stem, however, from children's feelings of inadequacy when faced with academic tasks that require these skills or from deficits in language that interfere with social competence. Children who demonstrate depressive symptoms also are found to have language difficulties that reflect inadequate verbal pragmatic skills, such as difficulties producing coherent and relevant utterances, describing internal emotional states, distinguishing between old and new information, and sequencing events over time [29,33]. Furthermore, there is evidence that children rated as shy and withdrawn by their teachers have problems with communication that go beyond timidity and are related to poor structural language and pragmatic language [34].

Anxiety disorder may be diagnosed when anxieties are intense or continue longer than expected. Specific anxiety disorders are distinguished on the basis of the focus of the anxiety. Most relevant to this discussion are separation anxiety and social phobia. Although anxiety, like depression, can influence academic and social functioning, it also may be a reaction to problems communicating in school and social settings. Moreover, if an anxiety disorder is accompanied by an unidentified LI, deficits in language potentially can affect the efficacy of treatments, where language is important for identifying and expressing thoughts or emotions, directing behavior, challenging or modifying anxious self-talk (by saying to oneself that you can handle the situation), or engaging in control of anxious behavior.

Children who have separation anxiety disorder have excessive anxiety when placed in situations where they are separated from an attachment figure or from home. Problems with separation can be exacerbated by LI. If children cannot express their feelings or worries accurately, if they cannot understand others, or if they have difficulty negotiating separations verbally, their already intense anxiety over the separation may be intensified.

The central feature of social phobia is a marked and persistent fear of acting in an embarrassing way in a social or performance situation. This can manifest as fear of social activities and situations, such as speaking or reading in public, initiating or maintaining conversations, and talking to authority figures [35]. In classrooms, children who have social phobia may seem to dislike certain subjects (eg, those that require reading or speaking in front of the class or social activities). There is overlap between these behavioral manifestations and those found in children who have LI. Children who have LI also may be reluctant to speak in class or may be placed in situations where their poor language and communication skills are noticed. Similar to children who have LI, children who have social phobia often have few friends. In school situations, teachers describe them as "loners." In fact, children diagnosed as having LI at 5 years have been found to exhibit social phobia as adolescents [36].

Prognosis for language impairment

Literature on the long-term outcomes for children who have LI and co-occurring psychopathology indicates that even children who have mild LI or children who have had treatment continue to experience difficulties with language-related tasks into adolescence and adulthood [1]. Some children identified with LI in preschool and whose LI seems to resolve before school entry (based on performance on tests of vocabulary and grammar) continue to show deficits in reading-related skills in adolescence. This suggests that children who have mild or resolved LI may not encounter problems with language-related activities until language demands on academic and social life increase in adolescence [1]. Identification and treatment of language difficulties are important at this age, as research suggests a direct link between unidentified LI in adolescence and juvenile delinquency [37,38].

Children who have deficits in multiple areas of language and whose LI continues beyond the preschool years are at the greatest risk for learning problems and social-emotional difficulties. Although learning difficulties in language-related skills, such as reading, are expected, LI also can be associated with deficits in mathematics [1]. This makes sense since social communication, particularly between caregiver and child, supports the development of numeric skills from later infancy onward [39]. Moreover, numeric cognition is learned and conveyed via oral communication.

With respect to social-emotional difficulties, a review of the literature indicates that as children who have LI move into adulthood, they are at continued risk for psychiatric disorder and poor overall social functioning [1]. This risk increases rather than decreases with time, even in children whose language functioning seems to improve.

Longitudinal research indicates that some types of LI are more likely to increase the risk for subsequent language and psychiatric problems [1]. The prognosis for children who have receptive LI is especially poor. Receptive language problems are subtle and can be more difficult to detect than expressive language problems. Even speech-language pathologists may experience difficulty detecting receptive language problems until a formal assessment is done. This emphasizes the need for routine examination, as problems with understanding language negatively affect learning and social interactions and also how adults view some behaviors (eg, inability to follow directions may be seen as intentional misbehavior) and children's view of themselves and their self-concept.

Longitudinal research can underestimate the long-term difficulties that children who have LI experience, because LI is complex and the outcome may depend on the severity of the presenting complaint and how a LI influences and is influenced by other aspects of development. Moreover, most longitudinal research focuses on children who have deficits in structural language. There are limited data on other aspects of language in children who have LI and co-occurring psychopathology. Longitudinal studies tend to focus on children's language-behavior profile at specific points in time. This ignores the ongoing interactions between children and their changing environment, which might influence the developmental trajectory of LI and its relationship to psychopathology. Furthermore, there is less research on language during adolescence, a time when the integrative aspects of language become especially important and have an impact on multiple facets of learning and behavior.

Language impairment and social-emotional disorder

Although the overlap between LI and social-emotional disorders has come to be appreciated, language problems as a possible contributor to psychopathology still is not commonly considered. To understand better how language might contribute to social-emotional disorder, it is helpful to look at their relationship in different developmental periods.

The few studies that have investigated preschoolers who have LI seen in mental health settings indicate that LI is associated with significant social-emotional disorder and that treating a LI is an important component of early intervention [9]. One study showed that children who have co-occurring LI and social-emotional disorder benefited from an intensive day treatment program and that these children made greater gains than children referred for social-emotional problems alone [40]. Moreover, gains in language functioning preceded behavioral gains, supporting the contribution of LI to psychopathology.

A large proportion of school-aged children referred to mental health settings (and to special classes for behavioral or emotional problems) have LI [2,27,28]. For some of these children, their LI was not identified or even suspected until a routine systematic research assessment was done. A question, then, is whether or not these children are different in some way from the children who already are identified as having LI. It seems that some children's language problems may be overlooked because their expressive language deficits are mild [41]. Severe expressive language deficits are easier to detect than mild expressive or receptive language deficits, which are more subtle and easier to attribute to other causes (eg, behavioral). Another reason language problems can be overlooked is if they are accompanied by relatively mild academic problems [28]. In this case, the emotional or behavioral problems could be more salient and mild underachievement more easily attributable to psychosocial factors rather than learning or language difficulties.

The majority of studies that investigate how LI and social-emotional disorder are linked in school-aged children tend to focus on structural language. The most consistent association of social-emotional disorder is with receptive LI and with structural language problems that are pervasive [9]. More recently, narrative discourse has been examined in children who have LI and social-emotional disorder. This is important because mental health professionals often perceive children's problems with communication as a consequence of social-emotional disturbance. Such problems include difficulties formulating and expressing thoughts; sounding incoherent because of the unclear and ambiguous way that people, objects, and events are referred to; and struggling to answer or providing only brief answers to direct questions. These symptoms, however, also could be interpreted as discourse deficits that are part of LI. The discourse of children who have LI and social-emotional disorder seems to have a unique profile [12]. As expected, these children have deficits exhibited by children who have LI and by children who have social-emotional disorder but they also demonstrate some distinct discourse problems, including difficulties with pronominal reference and making causal connections. Pronominal reference allows listeners to follow the people in a story from one context to another (eg, "Rob went to a movie. He went home right after."), and causal connections join events together in a logical manner ("I am sad because I had a nightmare"). Consequently, there could be an alternative explanation for some of the discourse difficulties of children in classrooms or in clinical or therapeutic settings, such as problems expressing their thoughts concisely. Rather than attributing these difficulties solely to emotional or behavioral factors, broader language deficits should be considered as an alternative explanation in some cases. Clinical or therapeutic settings are contexts that require language on demand, because children often are asked to formulate responses to specific questions (on topics often chosen by a therapist) in a timely manner. This is not an ideal type of communicative setting for children who have LI.

Remarkably little is known about the language characteristics of adolescents who have LI; however, research shows that adolescents' persisting language problems affect their personal relationships, academic success, choice of vocational and professional careers, and subsequent earning ability [24,25,42,43]. In adolescence, LI presumed to be resolved may re-emerge, as more complex higher-order language demands increase. Moreover, for some youth, LI may appear for the first time, again because of the increased demands on language during adolescence. Little research has examined LI and psychopathology in adolescents specifically, although juvenile delinquency is linked to deficits in basic skills, such as speaking and writing abilities. It is possible that early language problems are compounded when youth feel alienated from the mainstream and become less likely to continue in their attempts to achieve given the unrewarding outcome. The alienation is exacerbated because youth who have LI are more apt to be rejected by their peers and, as a consequence, delinquent behavior may serve as an alternate means of obtaining social status for some. Teachers and parents are less likely to be supportive of youth who have a "bad attitude" or rebel against societal norms.

There is a small body of research that directly links juvenile delinquency with adolescent LI [37,38]. This research indicates that delinquent youth have poorer language skills; they produce less complex language, have difficulties sequencing ideas, and exhibit deficits in pragmatic language. This same research indicates that only a small proportion of these youth receive special education services during their school years before their involvement with the law, and if services are provided they tend to be for learning disabilities (which do not necessarily address language needs) or behavioral disorders rather than LI.

On a more positive side, a review of literature examining long-term effects of reading disability into adolescence shows that childhood behavioral problems do not necessarily lead to high rates of antisocial behavior or social-emotional problems [1]. Factors, such as severity of difficulties and the context in which problems emerged, influenced outcomes; those children who received support and encouragement at home, had specialized attention at school, and who chose environments as adults consistent with their strengths and weaknesses did better. Although this research focused on children who had reading disabilities, it is likely that the majority of children also had LI. These findings provide general guidelines for promoting the mental health of children who have LI and emphasize the need for more systematic screening of children whose problems with learning and communication are attributed to social and emotional factors.

Models of language impairment

As yet, there is no comprehensive model that explains the diverse deficits in children who have LI and that addresses the interrelation of language, cognition, social cognition, and psychopathology. There is increasing interest in examining the cognitive correlates of LI, social cognition, and psychiatric disorder (in particular conduct disorder and ADHD) [31]. Recently, researchers have suggested that children who have LI might suffer a general limitation in their information processing capacity, which helps explain their linguistic and nonlinguistic deficits [6]. An attractive feature of this account of LI is that it allows language to be examined in relation to other developmental domains and demonstrates that LI does not exist in a vacuum. A recent study supports this view but indicates that children who have LI actually may have problems using their available processing capacity efficiently in the service of language tasks because of deficits in executive function [5]. A similar process could apply in explaining the interrelations between language, cognition, social cognition, and psychopathology in these children.

Summary

A large proportion of children who have LI have a comorbid psychiatric disorder or some type of social-emotional problem. The relationship is complex and likely involves other factors (including cognitive, social-cognitive, social-emotional, and affect and behavior regulation) that interact with experience and over development. Depending on the developmental task children are struggling with at a particular time, the LI or the social-emotional problem may seem more salient than the other. As such, a life-span approach to understanding the developmental trajectory for the interface of LI and social-emotional disorder is essential for theoretic and practical purposes. Communication begins in the first days of life, and ongoing transactions between physical and interpersonal environments and other domains of development can set a course that leads to different outcomes, some positive and others less so. Even a mild deficit in language ultimately can have a significant long-term impact, depending on its interaction with experience at critical developmental turning points. Thus, those who work with children and adolescents should consider that there might be associated conditions, such as LI, that interact with or contribute to the presenting problem in significant ways.

Key points

- The relationship between LI and social-emotional disorders is complex, and it is not always possible to make a clear differential diagnosis. Sometimes one disorder seems to lead to secondary symptomatology. In other cases, LI may be an inherent part of social-emotional disorder.
- Evidence points toward the long-term persistence of LI, even among those whose language problems seem to be resolved. For some children, LI may appear only later in childhood and adolescence, when language demands on academic tasks and social life increase.
- Research spanning the years from preschool through adolescence indicates that LI consistently is related to social-emotional disorder. Moreover, a large proportion of children presenting for mental health services and placed in classes for children who have social-emotional problems have LI left unidentified or unsuspected unless a formal assessment is done. These children are as much at risk for language, communication, cognitive, and social-cognitive problems as children whose LI is identified.

- In mental health settings, on the surface, there are many similarities in children's presenting problems. These problems may be associated with markedly different underlying conditions, however, some of which are related to language and associated impairments. Whether or not this is the case can be determined only if a thorough multifocused assessment is done.

References

[1] Cohen NJ. Developmental language disorders. In: Howlin P, Udwin O, editors. Outcomes in developmental and genetic disorders. Cambridge (UK): Cambridge University Press; 2002. p. 26–55.

[2] Camarata SM, Hughes CA, Ruhl KL. Mild/moderate behaviorally disordered students: a population at risk for language disorders. Lang Speech Hear Serv Sch 1988;19:191–200.

[3] Cantwell DP, Baker L. Psychiatric and developmental disorders in children with communication disorder. Washington, DC: American Psychiatric Press; 1991.

[4] Leonard LB. Children with specific language impairment. Cambridge (MA): MIT Press; 1998.

[5] Im-Bolter N, Johnson J, Pascual-Leone J. Processing limitations in children with specific language impairment: the role of executive function. Child Dev 2006;77:1822–41.

[6] Johnston JR. Cognitive abilities of children with language impairment. In: Watkins RV, Rice ML, editors. Specific language impairments in children. Baltimore (MD): Paul H. Brookes; 1994. p. 107–21.

[7] Fensen L, Dale P, Reznick S, et al. MacArthur-Bates communicative development inventory. Baltimore (MD): Paul H. Brookes Publishing; 1993.

[8] Wetherby AM, Prizant BM. Communication and symbolic behavior scales. Baltimore (MD): Paul H. Brookes Publishing; 1993.

[9] Cohen NJ. Language impairment and psychopathology in infants, children, and adolescents. London: Sage Publications; 2001.

[10] Stanovich KE, Siegel LS. Phenotypic performance profiles of children with reading disabilities: a regression-based test of the phonological-core variable-difference model. J Educ Psychol Psychology 1994;86:24–53.

[11] Montgomery JW. Understanding the language difficulties of children with specific language impairment: does verbal working memory matter? Am J Speech Lang Pathol 2002;11:77–91.

[12] Vallance DD, Im N, Cohen NJ. Discourse deficits associated with psychiatric disorders and with language impairments in children. J Child Psychol Psychiatry 1999;40:693–704.

[13] Nippold M, Uhden L, Schwartz I. Proverb explanation through the lifespan: a developmental study of adolescents and adults. J Speech Lang Hear Res 1997;40:245–53.

[14] Norbury CF. Factors supporting idiom comprehension in children with communication disorders. J Speech Lang Hear Res 2004;47:1179–93.

[15] Sroufe LA, Rutter M. The domain of developmental psychopathology. Child Dev 1984;55: 17–29.

[16] Cicchetti D, Beeghly M. An organizational approach to the study of Down syndrome: contributions to an integrative theory of development. In: Cicchetti D, Beeghly M, editors. Children with Down syndrome: a developmental perspective. Cambridge (MA): Cambridge University press; 1990. p. 29–62.

[17] Marton K, Abramoff B, Rosenzweig S. Social cognition and language in children with specific language impairment (SLI). J Commun Disord 2005;38:143–62.

[18] Zadeh ZY, Im-Bolter N, Cohen NJ. Social cognition and externalizing psychopathology: an investigation of the mediating role of language. J Abnorm Child Psychol, in press.

[19] Barkley R. Behavioral inhibition, sustained attention, and executive functions: constructing a unifying theory of ADHD. Psychol Bull 1997;121:65–94.

[20] Blake J, Myszczyszyn D, Jokel A. Spontaneous measures of morphosyntax in specifically language-impaired children. Appl Psycholinguist 2004;25:29–41.
[21] National Institute on Deafness and Other Communicative Disorders. National strategic research plan for language and language impairments, balance and balance disorders, and voice disorders. NIH Publication No. 97–3217. Bethesda (MD): National Institute on Deafness and Other Communicative Disorders; 1995.
[22] Beitchman JH, Nair R, Clegg M, et al. Prevalence of speech and language disorders in 5-year-old kindergarten children in the Ottawa-Carleton region. J Speech Hear Disord 1986;51: 98–110.
[23] Tomblin JB, Records NL, Zhang X. A system for the diagnosis of specific language impairment in kindergarten children. J Speech Lang Hear Res 1996;39:1284–94.
[24] Beitchman JH, Wilson B, Brownlie EB, et al. Long-term consistency in speech/language profiles: I. Developmental and academic outcomes. J Am Acad Child Adolesc Psychiatry 1996; 35:804–14.
[25] Beitchman JH, Wilson B, Brownlie EB, et al. Long-term consistency in speech/language profiles: II. Behavioral, emotional, and social outcomes. J Am Acad Child Adolesc Psychiatry 1996;35:815–25.
[26] American Psychiatric Association. Diagnostic and statistical manual of mental disorders (DSM IV). 4th (revised) edition. Washington, DC: American Psychiatric Association; 2000.
[27] Cohen NJ, Vallance DD, Barwick M, et al. The interface between ADHD and language impairment: an examination of language, achievement, and cognitive processing. J Child Psychol Psychiatry 2000;41:353–62.
[28] Cohen NJ, Barwick MA, Horodezky NB, et al. Language, achievement, and cognitive processing in psychiatrically disturbed children with previously identified and unsuspected language impairments. J Child Psychol Psychiatry 1998;39:865–77.
[29] Audet L, Ripich D. Psychiatric disorders and discourse problems. In: Ripich DN, Creaghead NA, editors. School discourse problems. San Diego (CA): Singular Publishing; 1994. p. 191–227.
[30] Kaler SR, Kopp C. Compliance and comprehension in very young toddlers. Child Dev 1990; 61:1997–2003.
[31] Moffitt TE. Neuropsychology of conduct disorders. Dev Psychopathol 1993;5:135–51.
[32] Gilmour J, Hill B, Place M, et al. Social communication deficits in conduct disorder: a clinical and community survey. J Child Psychol Psychiatry 2004;45:967–78.
[33] Baltaxe CAM, Simmons JQ. Communication deficits in preschool children with psychiatric disorders. Semin Speech Lang 1988;9:81–91.
[34] Donaghue ML, Hartis D, Cole D. Research on interactions among oral language and emotional behavioral disorders. In: Rogers-Adkinson DL, Griffith PL, editors. Communication disorders and children with psychiatric and behavioral disorders. San Diego (CA): Singular Publishing; 1999. p. 69–98.
[35] Beidel DC, Turner TL, Morris TL. Psychopathology of childhood social phobia. J Am Acad Child Adolesc Psychiatry 1999;38:630–46.
[36] Beitchman JH, Wilson B, Johnson CJ, et al. Fourteen-year follow-up of speech/language impaired and control children: psychiatric outcome. J Am Acad Child Adolesc Psychiatry 2001;40:75–82.
[37] Sanger D, Moore-Brown B, Alt E. Advancing discussion on communication and violence. Communication Disorders Quarterly 2000;22:43–8.
[38] Sanger D, Moore-Brown B, Magnuson G, et al. Prevalence of language problems among adolescent delinquents. Communications Disorders Quarterly 2001;23:17–26.
[39] Donlan C. The early numeracy of children with specific language impairments. In: Baroody AJ, Dowker A, editors. The development of arithmetic concepts and skills: constructing adaptive expertise. Mahwah (NJ): Lawrence Erlbaum; 2003. p. 337–58.
[40] Cohen NJ, Kolers N, Bradley S. Predictors of the outcome of treatment in a therapeutic preschool. J Am Acad Child Adolesc Psychiatry 1987;26:829–33.

[41] Cohen NJ, Davine M, Horodezky NB, et al. Unsuspected language impairment in psychiatrically disturbed children: prevalence and language and behavioral characteristics. J Am Acad Child Adolesc Psychiatry 1993;32:595–603.

[42] Snowling M, Bishop DVM, Stothard SE. Is preschool language impairment a risk factor for dyslexia in adolescence? J Child Psychol Psychiatry 2000;41:587–600.

[43] Stothard SE, Snowling MJ, Bishop DVM, et al. Language-impaired preschoolers: a follow-up into adolescence. J Speech Lang Hear Res 1998;41:407–18.

ELSEVIER
SAUNDERS

PEDIATRIC CLINICS
OF NORTH AMERICA

Pediatr Clin N Am 54 (2007) 543–561

Neuropsychology and Genetics of Speech, Language, and Literacy Disorders

Robin L. Peterson, MA[a],*, Lauren M. McGrath, MA[a],
Shelley D. Smith, PhD[b,c], Bruce F. Pennington, PhD[a,d]

[a]*Department of Psychology, University of Denver,
2155 South Race Street, Denver, CO 80208, USA*
[b]*Department of Pediatrics, University of Nebraska Medical Center,
985456 Nebraska Medical Center, Omaha, NE 68198-5456, USA*
[c]*Hattie B. Munroe Molecular Genetics, University of Nebraska Medical Center,
985456 Nebraska Medical Center, Omaha, NE 68198-5456, USA*
[d]*Developmental Neuropsychology Laboratory, University of Denver,
2155 South Race Street, Denver, CO 80208, USA*

This article provides an overview of the neuropsychology, neural substrates, and genetics of three disorders of language development: (1) developmental dyslexia, or reading disability (RD); (2) language impairment (LI); and (3) speech sound disorder (SSD). The three disorders are comorbid, and the authors review accumulating evidence for their overlap at the symptomatic, neuropsychologic, neural, and etiologic levels. The overlap is not complete, however, and researchers are still learning why, for example, some children have difficulties with speech sound production but not with reading. Of the three disorders, scientists know the most about RD across all the levels of analysis covered in this review, and the least about SSD. The amount of space dedicated to each disorder in this article reflects the current knowledge base of the field.

This work was supported by Grant No. HD049027 from the National Institute of Health and Human Development.
* Corresponding author.
E-mail address: rpeters6@du.edu (R.L. Peterson).

doi:10.1016/j.pcl.2007.02.009

pediatric.theclinics.com

Definitions and epidemiology

Current definitions of RD, LI, and SSD have two parts: (1) a diagnostic threshold and (2) a list of exclusionary conditions, which usually includes a peripheral sensory impairment (eg, deafness), a peripheral deficit in the vocal apparatus, acquired neurologic insults, environmental deprivation, and other more severe developmental disorders (such as autism or mental retardation). The first part of each definition concerns the central problem in the disorder. For RD, this problem lies in fluent or accurate printed word recognition. For LI, the defining problem concerns structural language, including syntax (grammar) and semantics (vocabulary), whereas for SSD the defining problem is in the ability to accurately and intelligibly produce the sounds of one's native language. In each case, setting a diagnostic threshold means imposing a somewhat arbitrary cutoff on a continuous variable (eg, Ref. [1]). A further issue has been whether the diagnostic cutoff should be drawn relative to age or IQ expectations for the particular ability involved. The logic of IQ-discrepant definitions is that they identify "pure" cases with a specific deficit, rather than a more general learning difficulty. The research literature generally has not supported the external validity of the distinction between age- and IQ-discrepancy definitions for either the underlying deficit or the kind of treatment that is helpful [2–4]. There is thus a growing consensus that age-referenced definitions are preferable, particularly for clinical purposes. Some research investigations may continue to benefit from an IQ discrepancy definition to identify the purest cases, however [5].

Prevalence estimates, of course, depend on definition. A commonly used cutoff for RD identifies 7% of the population by selecting those whose reading achievement is 1.5 standard deviations below the mean for age. An influential definition of LI requires performance on two language composites to fall below the tenth percentile; this definition identified 7.4% of an epidemiologic sample of kindergartners [6]. The prevalence of SSD declines sharply after the preschool period [7]. In an epidemiologic sample of 6-year-old children, 3.8% met criteria for SSD [8] compared with 15.6% of 3-year-old children [9]. These studies included only children making developmentally inappropriate speech errors; the prevalence is higher if children making errors considered developmentally appropriate that nonetheless interfere with intelligibility are included. All three disorders show a slight male predominance (approximately 1.5:1 [6,8,10]). Although there is widespread agreement that RD, LI, and SSD are all comorbid, specific comorbidity estimates vary widely depending on precise definitions, the age range studied, and the degree to which all three disorders (as opposed to only two) are accounted for. One consistent finding has been that children who have early language impairments are at high risk for later reading problems, with approximately 50% meeting criteria for RD [11,12]. In contrast, fewer children with isolated speech sound production difficulties meet full criteria for RD, although their literacy attainment may still lag behind that of appropriate controls [13,14].

Neuropsychology

Of the disorders considered in this article, researchers know the most about RD. This is largely because dyslexia is so well defined at the cognitive level of analysis. The cognitive analysis of dyslexia has provided both a fairly precise diagnostic phenotype and cognitive components of that phenotype. These cognitive components have proved useful as endophenotypes in genetic and neuroimaging studies. Although it might seem that science should start at lower levels of analysis, such as the etiologic or neural levels, understanding of complex behavioral disorders (including those considered in this article) generally relies on first establishing a sound neuropsychologic theory to define the behavioral phenotypes to tie to any putative neural substrates or genetic causes. Our understanding of SSD and LI across all levels of analysis becomes greatly enriched once we develop more complete neuropsychologic theories of these disorders.

Neuropsychology of reading disability

The ultimate goal of reading is reading comprehension. It turns out that a substantial proportion of the variation in reading comprehension can be accounted for by individual differences in the accuracy and speed of printed word recognition, especially in children [15]. According to the "simple view of reading" [16], reading comprehension (RC) equals the product of single word recognition (WR) and listening comprehension (LC). Empiric evidence has demonstrated that, in children, the product of WR and LC correlates highly with RC (0.84) [16]. The external validity of defining reading disability as characterized by deficits in accurate and fluent word recognition derives partly from the strong relationship of WR to RC. Of course, some children may have reading comprehension difficulties despite good WR skills because of impairments in LC. There is now evidence that such a group of children exists. They have been called "poor comprehenders" and are considered a diagnostically discrete category from RD (see Ref. [17] for a review.) Many poor comprehenders also meet criteria for LI [18], although most children who have LI have difficulties with RC resulting from deficits in both WR and LC. More recent research has also indicated that, as a group, children who have reading disability have problems with LC [19], indicating some phenotypic overlap between RD and LI. Further evidence for this phenotypic overlap comes from longitudinal studies demonstrating that preschoolers who later become RD show early deficits in syntax and semantics (eg, Ref. [20]). The notion that RD arises purely from WR deficits is therefore an oversimplification. This oversimplification allowed for many of the important recent discoveries about RD, however.

Word recognition can itself be broken down into two component written language skills, phonologic coding (PC), and orthographic coding (OC). PC refers to the ability to use knowledge of rule-like letter–sound correspondences to pronounce words that have never been seen before (usually measured by pseudoword reading), and OC refers to the use of word-specific patterns to aid in word recognition and pronunciation. Words that do not follow typical letter–sound correspondences (eg, *have* or *yacht*) must rely, at least in part, on OC to be recognized, as do homophones (eg, *rows* versus *rose*). A topic of ongoing debate in the adult and developmental literatures has been the extent to which successful PC and OC are achieved by separable cognitive mechanisms [21–23]. One question relevant to that debate is whether there are subtypes of RD that result from impairment to one mechanism or the other. This debate is beyond the scope of this article. The evidence is clear, however, that as a group, children who have RD are impaired at both PC and OC, and a common cause is supported by genetic studies showing that both deficits are linked to the same loci [24,25]. Further, the deficit in PC is generally considered more central because of extensive research documenting that, on the whole, individuals who have RD read pseudowords less accurately than even younger, normal readers matched on real word reading accuracy [26]. We argue that the great majority of children who have RD have difficulties with real word recognition resulting largely from PC deficits.

A complete neuropsychologic theory of RD must also specify the cognitive deficits that lead to phonologic coding difficulties. One family of tasks that has received particular attention measures phoneme awareness, an oral language skill that includes the ability to manipulate and attend to individual sounds in words. As an example of one kind of phoneme awareness task, the child is asked to "say 'fixed' without the '/k/'" with the correct answer being "fist." Individuals who have RD perform poorly on phoneme awareness tasks relative to both age-matched controls and younger, typically developing readers. Such tasks are among the best predictors of later reading ability, and phoneme awareness training positively influences later reading skill (see [27] for a recent review). Taken together, the evidence suggests that phoneme awareness plays a causal role in RD. This relationship presumably arises because the ability to map individual sounds onto letters—the defining characteristic of phonologic coding—relies on the ability to break spoken words apart into sounds and to attend to those sounds individually.

It now seems likely that both phonologic coding and phonologic awareness impairments in RD arise from lower-level deficits in the development of phonologic representations (ie, mental representations of individual speech sounds). Evidence for this view comes from the association of RD with poor performance on a wide variety of phonologic tasks, including phonologic memory, confrontational naming, and rapid naming [27]. These are all oral language tasks, buttressing the argument that RD is a language disorder. Further, children who have RD have difficulties with some speech perception tasks that do not require metalinguistic awareness [28,29].

Historical theories of RD postulated a basic deficit in visual processing and focused on the reversal errors commonly made by individuals who had RD, such as writing *b* for *d* or "was" for "saw" [30,31]. The simple visual theory of RD has been discredited for more than 25 years; Vellutino [32] demonstrated that such reversal errors in RD were restricted to print in one's own language, and were thus really linguistic rather than visual in nature. Several more current hypotheses also propose that RD results from a nonlinguistic, low-level sensory deficit. For example, the magnocellular hypothesis holds that RD results from difficulties with rapidly processing visually presented material [33]. The auditory hypothesis does not deny deficits in phonologic representations in RD, but posits that these deficits result from more basic, nonlinguistic, auditory processing problems [34,35]. (The auditory hypothesis was originally proposed to account for LI and is discussed later.) Indeed, RD participants have shown reliable group deficits on visual and auditory tasks. The argument for causality is damaged by a case-by-case inspection of data, however, which has consistently revealed that many RD participants do not have sensory deficits, whereas some control participants do (see Ref. [36] for a review). One interpretation is that RD sometimes co-occurs with more general sensory difficulties that are not the cause of the central phonologic coding deficit [36,37].

Neuropsychology of language impairment

A challenge to researchers studying the neuropsychology of LI has been the heterogeneity of the phenotype. At the symptomatic level, children's primary difficulties can range from expressive syntax to receptive vocabulary. Efforts to delineate reliable subtypes of LI have not met with great success, however, partly because subtypes based on symptom descriptions do not show adequate longitudinal stability [38]. The search for a core underlying deficit in LI has led to three competing proposals: the extended optional infinitive hypothesis, the phonologic memory hypothesis, and the auditory hypothesis. These hypotheses differ importantly in the specificity of the proposed impairment, and each is reviewed briefly later. We believe that current evidence best supports the phonologic memory hypothesis. Even this hypothesis is clearly incomplete, however, probably because any single core deficit will be inadequate to account for the full LI phenotype [39].

Of the three hypotheses, the extended optional infinitive proposal of Rice and colleagues [40] is the most specific; it posits that the core deficit in LI lies in the acquisition of a particular aspect of syntax. Evidence for this hypothesis is that children who have LI make characteristic errors in their expressive language. In English, they most notably have difficulties with the past tense, often substituting an unmarked form for a marked one (eg, "He walk there" in place of "He walked there.") This kind of error is made by typically developing children early in language acquisition, but children who have LI tend to use unmarked (or infinitive) forms much longer than even younger, typically developing children matched for overall language skill. Despite the elegance of this proposal, it faces two major challenges in trying to account for all cases of LI. First, it does not adequately explain the cross-linguistic data, which have shown that the syntactic forms causing the most difficulty for language-impaired children vary with their perceptual salience in different languages [41]. In English, for example, the past tense may be problematic partly because its marker ("–ed") is brief and often unstressed. Second, this proposal fails to explain why children who have LI perform poorly on a wide range of language tasks, including those that do not require syntactic competence [38]. The value of this marker may be in its persistence with age, making it an important endophenotype for genetic studies.

The phonologic memory hypothesis of LI holds that the core deficit lies in the ability to hold phonologic forms in working memory [42]. Phonologic memory is most often measured by asking children to repeat spoken lists of real words, such as numbers (digit span) or individual pseudowords (non-word repetition). This proposal is theoretically attractive because work with brain-damaged adults, second-language learners, and typically developing children has converged in highlighting a role for phonologic memory in language learning, particularly vocabulary acquisition [43]. Further, a recent computational model demonstrated that phonologic deficits caused impaired syntax learning [44]. Phonologic memory impairment does seem to be a robust endophenotype for LI. Phonologic memory deficits are heritable and correlate significantly with degree of language difficulty in individuals who have LI [45]. Further, phonologic memory deficits persist even in individuals whose broader language problems have resolved [46]. The phonologic memory hypothesis is unlikely to fully account for LI, however, because children who have RD and SSD also show phonologic memory deficits, often in the face of spared broader language function. To account for this pattern of findings, Bishop and Snowling [47] proposed a two by two classification for developmental language disorders based on the presence or absence of (1) phonologic deficits and (2) broader language deficits, including semantics and syntax. According to this scheme, RD is associated with phonologic deficits only, whereas LI is associated with deficits on both dimensions. Because broader language deficits are the defining symptom in LI, however, this classification scheme remains descriptive. A neuropsychologic theory must specify the cognitive components that underlie these deficits.

Finally, the auditory hypothesis of LI is the least specific because it posits that a nonlinguistic sensory impairment leads to both phonologic and broader language difficulties in LI. This hypothesis was developed in the 1970s by Tallal and Piercy [48] and in more recent years has been extended to RD (see previous discussion). Early studies demonstrated that children who had LI had specific difficulty discriminating rapidly presented nonspeech sounds, which presumably led to problems processing certain aspects of the speech stream. Later studies found that despite group differences, many children who have LI do not have auditory deficits, whereas many typically developing children do [49]. Further, there is little evidence that the auditory impairments described in these studies are heritable [45]. Because LI is partly heritable, this finding is problematic for the argument that deficits in the discrimination of rapid auditory stimuli are the sole cause of the disorder. It remains possible that auditory deficits of an environmental cause significantly complicate language development in children already at genetic risk for LI [45].

Neuropsychology of speech sound disorder

SSD was originally considered a disorder of generating oral-motor programs, and children who had speech sound impairments were said to have "functional articulation disorder" [38]. A careful analysis of error patterns has rendered a pure motor deficit unlikely as a full explanation for the disorder, however. For example, children who have SSD sometimes produce a sound correctly in one context but incorrectly in another. If children were unable to execute particular motor programs, then we might expect that most of their errors would take the form of phonetic distortions arising from an approximation of that motor program. The most common errors in children who have SSD are substitutions of phonemes, not distortions [41]. Further, a growing body of research is demonstrating that children who have SSD show deficits on a range of phonologic tasks, including phoneme awareness and phonologic memory [50–53]. Although it remains possible that a subgroup of children have speech sound difficulties primarily because of motor impairments, it now seems likely that most children who have SSD have a type of language disorder that primarily affects phonologic development. There is thus a puzzle to be resolved: if RD, LI, and SSD are all associated with phonologic impairments, why is their overlap not complete? One possibility is that phonologic deficits are a shared risk factor for all three disorders, with additional risk factors specific to each disorder [39]. For example, work in our laboratory showed that RD and SSD were associated with similar deficits in phoneme awareness and phonologic memory, but only RD was additionally associated with impairments in rapid naming [51,54].

Neural substrates

Anatomic findings

Evidence for structural abnormalities in the brains of individuals who have RD or LI has come from postmortem studies and MRI. To date, there is little research on the neuroanatomy of SSD. Interpretation of the RD and LI results is complicated because definitions of the disorders vary across studies, and many studies have not adequately addressed the question of co-morbidity. This confound can be seen in the pioneering work of Galaburda and colleagues, who reported a series of postmortem findings in individuals who had severe reading difficulties. One group of findings concerned histo-logic anomalies, including abnormally-sized cells, and ectopias and dyspla-sias presumed to result from failures of neural migration. Overall, these anomalies were more common in RD than control brains, particularly in perisylvian regions and in parts of the thalamus. A second group of post-mortem findings related to the planum temporale, a region of the superior temporal gyrus (STG) implicated in auditory and language processing. Most typically developing individuals show an asymmetry of this structure, with larger left hemisphere than right hemisphere volumes, whereas brains of several reading-disabled individuals showed symmetry [55,56]. Although this result has most often been assumed to relate to RD, it is likely that many of the individuals studied by Galaburda and colleagues would have also met criteria for language impairment [47]. In fact, symmetric plana tem-porale and perisylvian histologic anomalies have since been associated with LI [57,58].

More recent MRI studies have suggested that reduced or reversed pla-num temporale asymmetry is indeed more likely to be associated with LI than with RD. Although two early MRI studies supported the absence of a normal leftward asymmetry in RD, there have since been numerous fail-ures to replicate this finding and some reports of greater leftward asymmetry for individuals who have RD than controls [59]. In contrast, abnormal asymmetry of the planum temporale (or of the STG, which includes this structure) has been reported somewhat more consistently in the LI literature [57,60–63] (but see [64,65]). In one study that directly compared children who had RD to children who had LI, only the group that had LI had sym-metric plana temporale [62].

Another brain region that has garnered attention in the RD and LI liter-atures is the inferior frontal gyrus (IFG), which includes Broca's area, long known as a critical region for language production. This structure also shows a leftward asymmetry in most typically developing individuals, whereas studies have reported reduced or reversed asymmetry in LI [60,64]. De Fosse and colleagues [64] found that reduced leftward asymme-try correlated with lower verbal IQ. Findings for RD have been similar. For example, Brown and colleagues [66] reported gray matter decreases in the left IFG in individuals who had RD, whereas Robichon and colleagues [67] found an abnormal rightward asymmetry of the IFG in RD that corre-lated with pseudoword reading performance. It is thus possible that IFG ab-normalities confer risk for language impairment and reading disability.

Both disorders have also been associated with more widespread neural differences. RD researchers have reported abnormalities in many parts of the temporal lobes, in perisylvian regions of the parietal lobes, and in the cerebellum (see Ref. [68] for a review). LI researchers have reported differences across frontal, temporal, parietal, and subcortical regions [47]. Further, there have been some reports of total cerebral volume reduction in both RD [69,70] and LI [62,71]. In a direct comparison of children who had RD to children who had LI, however, volume reduction seemed specific to LI [62]. Furthermore, another study by the same research group reported that cerebral volume did not correlate with symptom measures that are central to RD (eg, pseudoword reading) but did correlate with measures more central to LI, such as oral comprehension [72].

Two exciting recent studies of RD participants used diffusion tensor imaging and reported disturbances in the white matter tracts connecting anterior and posterior perisylvian regions [73,74]. Similar techniques have yet to be used in LI samples and should be fruitful for future research.

In summary, structural findings in RD and LI have most often implicated left hemisphere perisylvian regions involved in skilled reading and language, although findings are by no means limited to these regions. The commonalities in structural findings for LI and RD are likely to be both meaningful (because some brain differences are probably shared by the disorders) and artifactual (because studies have not carefully controlled for comorbidity). Future studies should compare children who have only one of the disorders, both disorders, or neither (controls).

We are not aware of any studies that have specifically examined neuroanatomic correlates of SSD using a precisely defined phenotype. In-depth study of one British family, referred to as the KE family, has produced findings that could help guide future research. About half the KE family members are affected with a general language deficit impacting grammar and expressive language and a severe speech production disorder that significantly impairs intelligibility [75,76]. Affected members of the KE family thus meet criteria for LI and SSD, although it is not clear that they are representative of the larger population of individuals who have speech and language disorders. Their speech difficulty is often described as a verbal apraxia, a label that implies their articulation difficulties arise from impairments in sequencing oral-motor movements. It is possible that verbal apraxia is a subtype of SSD that is etiologically distinct from a more common, phonologically based subtype. MRI findings in the KE family indicated bilateral abnormalities in the basal ganglia, especially the caudate nucleus, and in the left IFG and premotor areas of affected family members [77]. Left caudate volume correlated with performance on a task of oral praxis, suggesting that this brain region in particular may relate to affected family members' articulation difficulties.

Functional findings

Several investigations have attempted to further elucidate the neural bases of RD by examining brain function during reading and language tasks using positron emission tomography (PET) and functional MRI (fMRI).

A smaller body of literature has investigated brain function in LI, and again there is almost no work on SSD. As in the anatomic literature, the comorbidity of these disorders has rarely been carefully addressed. Interpretation of functional results is further limited in studies that use a case-control design but do not equate performance across the two groups (see Ref. [78]). In these cases, it is not clear whether the neural differences are a cause or a result of impaired performance.

Functional neuroimaging studies of reading and language tasks have identified aberrant activation patterns in RD participants across a distributed set of left hemisphere sites, including many of the same regions implicated by the anatomic literature (see [78,79] for reviews). The most common findings have been reduced activation of left occipitotemporal and temporoparietal regions. Findings in the region of the left IFG have been mixed, with several studies reporting increased activation in RD, whereas others have reported decreased activation. Both task and participant characteristics likely contribute to the variability in findings. For example, increased IFG activity in RD has most often emerged in the context of reading aloud [78]. In silent reading or other language tasks, decreased activity in this region is more likely among the most impaired readers [80]. A common interpretation of the full pattern of results is that decreased occipitotemporal activity corresponds to deficits in word recognition processes (ie, OC), decreased temporoparietal activity corresponds to phonologic processing difficulties, and increased IFG activity relates to compensatory processes. Notably, few studies have equated performance across RD and control groups. This limitation particularly complicates the interpretation of temporoparietal findings, which (to date) have emerged only in the context of group performance differences [78].

Fewer studies have investigated the functional brain correlates of LI. One PET study compared brain activation in two affected members of the KE family to four normal controls [76]. The nature of the task used (word repetition minus a baseline articulation condition) meant that the results may relate more to the family's language impairment than to their speech difficulties. Affected family members showed aberrant activation patterns (some overactivation and some underactivation) across a widely distributed set of left hemisphere sites, including IFG, angular gyrus, motor and premotor areas, and caudate nucleus. Two more recent studies have used fMRI to examine brain function in LI outside the KE family. Hugdahl and colleagues [81] used a passive listening task that activated bilateral superior temporal gyrus (STG) and middle temporal gyrus (MTG) in control subjects. Activation for five individuals who had LI (all from one Finnish family) were similar to the control group, but smaller and weaker, particularly in the region of the superior temporal sulcus and MTG. Using a verbal working memory task, another research group found that children who had LI tended to have reduced activation across several left hemisphere sites, including the IFG, parietal regions, and the precentral sulcus [82]. One of the most exciting findings from this paper relied on a correlational analysis to examine the extent to which groups tended to coactivate different brain regions (possibly relating to their degree of anatomic connectivity.) Compared with the control group, the LI group showed less coactivation between STG and IFG, but more parietal–frontal and parietal–STG coactivation. Unfortunately, however, this study did not equate in-scanner performance across groups.

Taken together, the structural and functional neuroimaging literatures in RD and LI are beginning to implicate many of the brain regions involved in skilled reading and language—notably including the STG, the IFG, and temporoparietal regions. Researchers have just begun to explore how differences in the connectivity among these regions may relate to reading and language problems. To date, we have little understanding of how the neural substrates of RD and LI relate to each other and virtually no knowledge of the brain bases of SSD.

Genetics

Genetics of reading

There is convergence across different genetic methodologies that all three of the disorders considered in this article are partly heritable. Again, our knowledge of RD is deeper and has a longer history than our knowledge of the other two disorders, particularly SSD. The cognitive dissection of RD described previously proceeded hand in hand with decades of work demonstrating that RD and its cognitive components are familial and heritable [83] and are linked to several quantitative trait loci (QTLs) across the genome [84]. Seven replicated QTLs have been identified on 1p34-p36 (DYX8), 2p11-16 (DYX3), 3p12-q13 (DYX5), 6p21.3-22 (DYX2), 15q15-21 (DYX1), 18p11 (DYX6), and Xq27.3 (DYX9). Two additional genetic loci for RD are included on the most recent Human Gene Nomenclature Committee list (www.gene.ucl.ac.uk/nomenclature/). These are on 6q13-q16 (DYX4 [85]) and 11p15 (DYX7 [86]). There are currently nine genetic risk loci for RD, but two of these need additional replication to be convincing. This linkage work has now been followed by the initial identification of four candidate genes in three of these linkage regions: 3p12-q13 (ROBO1), 6p21.3-22 (DCDC2 and KIAA0319), and 15q15-21 (DYX1C1, initially labeled as EKN1) (see [87,88] for reviews).

The first candidate gene to be identified was DYX1C1 [89], so it has been the target of the most replication attempts (six so far). Five of these failed to find any association between DYX1C1 variants and RD phenotypes [90–94], but one study by Wigg and colleagues [95] found an association in the opposite direction, such that the more common, non-risk alleles of the haplotype proposed by the original work of Taipale and colleagues [89] were associated with the phenotype. They also found a significant association with an additional SNP that was not tested by Taipale and colleagues [89]. More work is needed to confirm or reject this candidate gene.

The other three candidate genes, ROBO1 [96], DCDC2 [97], and KIAA0319 [98], were identified more recently and thus have been tested less for replication. The DCDC2 candidate was replicated by Schumacher and colleagues [99] and KIAA0319 by Paracchini and colleagues [100].

One of the most exciting aspects of the work on all four candidate genes is that the role of each in brain development has been studied in animal models. Research using RNAi technology found that shutting down the expression of DCDC2 [97], KIAA0319 [100], and DYX1C1 [101] interferes with neuronal migration, consistent with Galaburda's discovery of ectopias in the brains of individuals who had RD. ROBO1 is also known to be involved in brain development, specifically in axon pathfinding. Andrews and colleagues [102] genetically modified mice so that they were lacking ROBO1 completely (a ROBO1 knockout). Although the knockout mice died at birth, they demonstrated prenatal axonal tract defects and neuronal migration defects in the forebrain.

These results from animal models indicate that alterations in DYX1C1, DCDC2, KIAA0319, and ROBO1 could disrupt human brain development in a way that is consistent with what little is known about the neuropathology of RD [103]. But to really prove causation requires several more steps: (1) the functional or regulatory mutations in these particular genes have to be identified, (2) it has to be demonstrated that these particular mutations disrupt brain development in animal models, and, most difficult of all, (3) it has to be shown that humans who have a dyslexic phenotype and these mutations have similar disruptions in brain development. Thus far, no mutations have been identified in coding regions of any of the candidate genes, so it is likely that mutations involve regulatory regions that control the level of gene product produced, rather than a faulty protein. This theory is consistent with the milder impairment of RD compared with more severe cognitive deficits that typically result from absent or defective gene products. In sum, the identification of candidate genes for RD has taken us all the way from cognitive dissection to developmental neurobiology, so that we are now able to test specific hypotheses about how brain development is disrupted in this prevalent disorder. This work is now developing rapidly, so new insights about brain development in RD are likely. One particular issue for future research is that each gene has been implicated in global brain developmental processes, such as neural migration and axonal guidance. There is a puzzle to be unraveled: how can a disruption in global brain development result in a relatively specific phenotype?

Genetics of language impairment and speech sound disorder

One striking example of the role of genes in language development comes from the KE family. About half the members of this family are affected with a general speech and language impairment impacting, most notably, expressive language and articulation. Pedigree analysis revealed that the inheritance pattern was consistent with a single gene, autosomal dominant trait [104]. The gene responsible for this disorder was eventually localized to the long arm of chromosome 7 in the 7q31 region and subsequently identified as the FOXP2 gene [75,105]. The simple Mendelian transmission of this disorder in the KE family is a unique example, which is probably not representative of the larger population of individuals who have speech and language disorders [106].

Analysis of LI outside the KE family indicates that although the disorder is significantly heritable, its cause is typically more consistent with a complex disease model, in which multiple causative risk factors (genetic and environmental) interact to produce an eventual phenotype. Genomewide scans of multiple families affected by LI have not identified FOXP2 as a candidate gene. Instead, significant linkage has been reported to 13q21 (using various language phenotypes), 16q (using a phonologic memory phenotype), and 19q (again, with various phenotypes) [107–109]. None of these loci overlap with those identified for RD, but some of the positive linkage results with LI individuals used reading phenotypes [107,109]. At this point, it is unclear if the lack of overlap between RD and LI risk loci is attributable to a lack of power or a true null finding.

The etiology of SSD outside the KE family also seems consistent with the complex disease model, and we are accumulating knowledge about specific genetic risk factors involved. Again, the FOXP2 gene does not seem to be implicated in most cases, although mutations in this gene may play a role in the development of SSD in a small minority of cases—notably, among individuals who seem to fit a verbal apraxia subtype [110]. Two independent studies have investigated whether SSD shows linkage to known RD risk loci [111,112]. These studies reported possible linkage of SSD to chromosome 1p36 and significant linkage to 3p12-q13 (where ROBO1 is located), 6p21.3-22 (where DCDC2 and KIAA0319 are located) and 15q21 (where DYX1C1 is located). Recent attempts to replicate the 1p36, 6p21.3-22 and 15q21 loci in an independent SSD sample have been partially successful. There is preliminary evidence of replication of the 1p36 [113] and 6p22 loci (S Iyengar, personal communication, 2006). There is evidence for a possible replication of the 15q21 locus, although these results are ambiguous because the linkage peak is closer to genes associated with autism and Prader-Willi/Angelman Syndrome than the region associated with dyslexia/SSD [114].

That SSD and RD seem to share genetic risk factors is consistent with these disorders being comorbid and associated with impairments in phonologic processing. The failure (to date) to find clear evidence for shared genetic risk factors for LI and RD is puzzling—these disorders are also comorbid, and as we have seen, they overlap at the symptom, neuropsychologic, and brain levels. Further, longitudinal studies have demonstrated that children who have early language impairments are at much higher risk for later RD than are children who have isolated speech sound difficulties, a finding that suggests that the overlap between RD and SSD is partly attributable to the third variable of LI. A goal of future research will be to identify shared etiologic risk factors for RD and LI and to clarify the etiologic relationship of all three disorders.

Etiologic interactions

The heritability of all three disorders considered in this chapter is significantly less than 100%, a factor that points to the importance of environmental variables in their development. Such variables are likely to include home language and literacy environments and instructional quality (especially for RD), along with environmental events that have a more direct effect on biology (eg, lead poisoning or head injury). Unfortunately, few studies investigating main effects of such environmental variables on language development have used genetically sensitive designs. In addition to main effects of environment, it is likely that the disorders considered here are influenced by gene by environment (G × E) interactions. A recent study in our lab investigated G × E using measures of the home language and literacy environment in a sample of children who had SSD and their siblings. We tested for G × E at the two SSD/RD linkage peaks with the strongest evidence of linkage to speech phenotypes, 6p22 and 15q21. The interactions were tested using speech, language, and preliteracy phenotypes. Results showed four significant and trend-level G × E interactions at both the 6p22 and 15q21 locations across several phenotypes and home environmental measures [115]. The direction of the interactions was such that in enriched environments genetic risk factors substantially influenced the phenotype, whereas in less optimal environments genetic risk factors had less influence on the phenotype. This directionality of the interactions is consistent with the bioecological model of G × E [116]. This work is preliminary because these linkage-based methods are a step away from the ideal of using identified risk alleles to test for G × E [117,118]. As molecular genetics identifies specific risk alleles for RD, SSD, and LI, the field will be able to more rigorously test etiologic models that include G × E interactions.

Summary

We have provided a brief overview of the symptoms, neuropsychology, brain bases, and genetics of three common disorders of language development: reading disability, language impairment, and speech sound disorder. Across levels of analysis, our understanding of RD is the most advanced, but it is by no means complete. For all three disorders, future work is required to precisely identify etiologic risk factors (ie, specific risk alleles, specific environmental conditions) and to discover how these interact to produce particular brain differences and behavioral phenotypes. Because there is partial, but not complete, overlap of the three disorders, this work is likely to produce findings that are common to all three disorders along with findings unique to each. Ultimately, our understanding of typical and atypical language development will be enriched by research that investigates not only RD, LI, or SSD alone but also the relationships of these disorders to each other.

References

[1] Rodgers B. The identification and prevalence of specific reading retardation. Br J Educ Psychol 1983;53:369–73.

[2] Fletcher JM, Foorman BR, Shaywitz SE, et al. Conceptual and methodological issues in dyslexia research: a lesson for developmental disorders. In: Tager-Flusberg H, editor. Neurodevelopmental disorders. Cambridge (MA): The MIT Press; 1999. p. 271–305.

[3] Stuebing KK, Fletcher JM, LeDoux JM, et al. Validity of IQ-discrepancy classifications of reading disabilities: a meta-analysis. Am Educ Res J 2002;39:469–518.

[4] Silva PA, McGee R, Williams S. Some characteristics of 9-year-old boys with general reading backwardness or specific reading retardation. J Child Psychol Psychiatry 1985;26:407–21.

[5] Knopik VS, Smith SD, Cardon L, et al. Differential genetic etiology of reading component processes as a function of IQ. Behav Genet 2002;32:181–98.

[6] Tomblin JB, Records NL, Buckwalter P, et al. Prevalence of specific language impairment in kindergarten children. J Speech Lang Hear Res 1997;40:1245–60.

[7] Shriberg LD, Gruber FA, Kwiatkowski J. Developmental phonological disorders: III. Long-term speech-sound normalization. J Speech Hear Res 1994;37:1151–77.

[8] Shriberg LD, Tomblin JB, McSweeny JL. Prevalence of speech delay in 6-year-old children and comorbidity with language impairment. J Speech Lang Hear Res 1999;42:1461–81.

[9] Campbell TF, Dollaghan CA, Rockette HE, et al. Risk factors for speech delay of unknown origin in 3-year-old children. Child Dev 2003;74:346–57.

[10] Shaywitz SE, Shaywitz BA, Fletcher JM, et al. Prevalence of reading disability in boys and girls. Results of the Connecticut Longitudinal Study. JAMA 1990;264:998–1002.

[11] Catts HW, Fey ME, Tomblin JB, et al. A longitudinal investigation of reading outcomes in children with language impairments. J Speech Lang Hear Res 2002;45:1142–57.

[12] Snowling MJ, Bishop DVM, Stothard SE. Is preschool language impairment a risk factor for dyslexia in adolescence? J Child Psychol Psychiatry 2000;41:587–600.

[13] Bishop DV, Adams C. A prospective study of the relationship between specific language impairment, phonological disorders and reading retardation. J Child Psychol Psychiatry 1990;31:1027–50.

[14] Bird J, Bishop DVM, Freeman N. Phonological awareness and literacy development in children with expressive phonological impairments. J Speech Hear Res 1995;38:446–62.

[15] Perfetti CA. Reading ability. Oxford: Oxford University Press; 1985.

[16] Gough PB, Walsh MA. Chinese, phoenicians, and the orthographic cipher of English. In: Brady SA, Shankweiler DP, editors. Phonological processes in literacy: a tribute to Isabelle Y. Liberman. Hillsdale (NJ): Lawrence Erlbaum Associates, Inc; 1991. p. 199–209.

[17] Nation K. Children's reading comprehension difficulties. In: Snowling MJ, Hulme C, editors. The science of reading: a handbook. Oxford: Blackwell Publishing; 2005. p. 248–65.

[18] Nation K, Clarke P, Marshall CM, et al. Hidden language impairments in children: parallels between poor reading comprehension and specific language impairment? J Speech Lang Hear Res 2004;47:199–211.

[19] Keenan JM, Betjemann RS, Wadsworth SJ, et al. Genetic and environmental influences on reading and listening comprehension. J Res Read 2006;29:75–91.

[20] Scarborough HS. Very early language deficits in dyslexic children. Child Dev 1990;61:1728–43.

[21] Harm MW, Seidenberg MS. Phonology, reading acquisition, and dyslexia: insights from connectionist models. Psychol Rev 1999;106:491–528.

[22] Harm MW, Seidenberg MS. Computing the meanings of words in reading: cooperative division of labor between visual and phonological processes. Psychol Rev 2004;111:662–720.

[23] Jackson NE, Coltheart M. Routes to reading success and failure: toward an integrated cognitive psychology of atypical reading. New York: Psychology Press; 2001.

[24] Gayan J, Smith SD, Cherny SS, et al. Quantitative-trait locus for specific language and reading deficits on chromosome 6p. Am J Hum Genet 1999;64:157–64.

[25] Fisher SE, Marlow AJ, Lamb J, et al. A quantitative-trait locus on chromosome 6p influences different aspects of developmental dyslexia. Am J Hum Genet 1999;64:146–56.

[26] Rack JP, Snowling MJ, Olson RK. The nonword reading deficit in developmental dyslexia: a review. Reading Research Quarterly 1992;27:28–53.

[27] Vellutino FR, Fletcher JM, Snowling MJ, et al. Specific reading disability (dyslexia): what have we learned in the past four decades? J Child Psychol Psychiatry 2004;45:2–40.

[28] Boada R, Pennington BF. Deficient implicit phonological representations in children with dyslexia. J Exp Child Psychol 2006;35:153–93.

[29] Werker JF, Tees RC. Speech perception in severely disabled and average reading children. Can J Psychol 1987;41:48–61.

[30] Orton ST. Word-blindness in school children. Arch Neurol Psychiatry 1925;14:581–615.

[31] Orton ST. Reading, writing and speech problems in children. New York: W.W. Norton & Co, Inc. 1937.

[32] Vellutino FR. The validity of perceptual deficit explanations of reading disability: a reply to Fletcher and Satz. J Learn Disabil 1979;12:160–7.

[33] Stein J, Walsh V. To see but not to read; the magnocellular theory of dyslexia. Trends Neurosci 1997;20:147–52.

[34] Tallal P. Auditory temporal perception, phonics, and reading disabilities in children. Brain Lang 1980;9:182–98.

[35] Tallal P, Miller SL, Jenkins WM, et al. The role of temporal processing in developmental language-based learning disorders: research and clinical implications. In: Blachman BA, editor. Foundations of reading acquisition and dyslexia: implications for early intervention. Hillsdale (NJ): Lawrence Erlbaum Associates, Publishers; 1997. p. 49–66.

[36] Ramus F. Developmental dyslexia: specific phonological deficit or general sensorimotor dysfunction? Curr Opin Neurobiol 2003;13:212–8.

[37] Hulslander J, Talcott J, Witton C, et al. Sensory processing, reading, IQ, and attention. J Exp Child Psychol 2004;88:274–95.

[38] Bishop DVM. Uncommon understanding: development and disorders of language comprehension in children. East Sussex (UK): Psychology Press/Erlbaum (UK) Taylor & Francis; 1997.

[39] Pennington BF. From single to multiple deficit models of developmental disorders. Cognition 2006;101:385–413.

[40] Rice ML, Wexler K, Cleave PL. Specific language impairment as a period of extended optional infinitive. J Speech Hear Res 1995;38:850–63.

[41] Leonard LB. Phonological impairment. In: Fletcher P, MacWhinney B, editors. The handbook of child language. Oxford (UK): Blackwell; 1995. p. 573–602.

[42] Gathercole SE, Baddeley AD. Phonological memory deficits in language disordered children: is there a causal connection? Journal of Memory and Language 1990;29:336–60.

[43] Baddeley A, Gathercole S, Papagno C. The phonological loop as a language learning device. Psychol Rev 1998;105:158–73.

[44] Joanisse MF, Seidenberg MS. Phonology and syntax in specific language impairment: evidence from a connectionist model. Brain Lang 2003;86:40–56.

[45] Bishop DVM, Bishop SJ, Bright P, et al. Different origin of auditory and phonological processing problems in children with language impairment: evidence from a twin study. J Speech Lang Hear Res 1999;42:155–68.

[46] Stothard SE, Snowling MJ, Bishop DVM, et al. Language-impaired preschoolers: a follow-up into adolescence. J Speech Lang Hear Res 1998;41:407–18.

[47] Bishop DV, Snowling MJ. Developmental dyslexia and specific language impairment: same or different? Psychol Bull 2004;130:858–86.

[48] Tallal P, Piercy M. Developmental aphasia: impaired rate of nonverbal processing as a function of sensory modality. Neuropsychologia 1973;11:389–98.

[49] Bishop DVM, Carlyon RP, Deeks JM, et al. Auditory temporal processing impairment: neither necessary nor sufficient for causing language impairment in children. J Speech Lang Hear Res 1999;42:1295–310.

[50] Bird J, Bishop D. Perception and awareness of phonemes in phonologically impaired children. Eur J Disord Commun 1992;27:289–311.

[51] Raitano NA, Pennington BF, Tunick RA, et al. Pre-literacy skills of subgroups of children with speech sound disorders. J Child Psychol Psychiatry 2004;45:821–35.

[52] Kenney MK, Barac-Cikoja D, Finnegan K, et al. Speech perception and short-term memory deficits in persistent developmental speech disorder. Brain Lang 2006;96:178–90.

[53] Leitao S, Hogben J, Fletcher J. Phonological processing skills in speech and language impaired children. Eur J Disord Commun 1997;32:73–93.

[54] Tunick RA, Pennington BF, Boada R. Cofamiliality of speech sound disorder and reading disability, submitted for publication.

[55] Livingstone MS, Rosen GD, Drislane FW, et al. Physiological and anatomical evidence for a magnocellular defect in developmental dyslexia. Proc Natl Acad Sci U S A 1991;88:7943–7.

[56] Galaburda AM, Menard MT, Rosen GD. Evidence for aberrant auditory anatomy in developmental dyslexia. Proc Natl Acad Sci U S A 1994;91:8010–3.

[57] Cohen M, Campbell R, Yaghmai F. Neuropathological abnormalities in developmental dysphasia. Ann Neurol 1989;25:567–70.

[58] de Vasconcelos Hage SR, Cendes F, Montenegro MA, et al. Specific language impairment: linguistic and neurobiological aspects. Arq Neuropsiquiatr 2006;64:173–80.

[59] Eckert MA, Leonard CM. Structural imaging in dyslexia: the planum temporale. Ment Retard Dev Disabil Res Rev 2000;6:198–206.

[60] Gauger LM, Lombardino LJ, Leonard CM. Brain morphology in children with specific language impairment. J Speech Lang Hear Res 1997;40:1272–84.

[61] Jernigan TL, Hesselink JR, Sowell E, et al. Cerebral structure on magnetic resonance imaging in language- and learning-impaired children. Arch Neurol 1991;48:539–45.

[62] Leonard CM, Lombardino LJ, Walsh K, et al. Anatomical risk factors that distinguish dyslexia from SLI predict reading skill in normal children. J Commun Disord 2002;35:501–31.

[63] Plante E, Swisher L, Vance R, et al. MRI findings in boys with specific language impairment. Brain Lang 1991;41:52–66.

[64] De Fosse L, Hodge SM, Makris N, et al. Language-association cortex asymmetry in autism and specific language impairment. Ann Neurol 2004;56:757–66.

[65] Preis S, Jancke L, Schittler P, et al. Normal intrasylvian anatomical asymmetry in children with developmental language disorder. Neuropsychologia 1998;36:849–55.

[66] Brown WE, Eliez S, Menon V, et al. Preliminary evidence of widespread morphological variations of the brain in dyslexia. Neurology 2001;56:781–3.

[67] Robichon F, Levrier O, Farnarier P, et al. Developmental dyslexia: atypical cortical asymmetries and functional significance. Eur J Neurol 2000;7:35–46.

[68] Eckert MA. Neuroanatomical markers for dyslexia: a review of dyslexia structural imaging studies. Neuroscientist 2004;10:362–71.

[69] Casanova MF, Araque J, Giedd J, et al. Reduced brain size and gyrification in the brains of dyslexic patients. J Child Neurol 2004;19:275–81.

[70] Phinney E, Pennington BF, Olson R, et al. Brain structure correlates of component reading processes: implications for reading disability. Cortex, in press.

[71] Trauner D, Wulfeck B, Tallal P, et al. Neurological and MRI profiles of children with developmental language impairment. Dev Med Child Neurol 2000;42:470–5.

[72] Leonard CM, Eckert MA, Lombardino LJ, et al. Anatomical risk factors for phonological dyslexia. Cereb Cortex 2001;11:148–57.

[73] Deutsch GK, Dougherty RF, Bammer R, et al. Children's reading performance is correlated with white matter structure measured by tensor imaging. Cortex 2005;41:354–63.

[74] Klingberg T, Hedehus M, Temple E, et al. Microstructure of temporo-parietal white matter as a basis for reading ability: evidence from diffusion tensor magnetic resonance imaging. Neuron 2000;25:493–500.

[75] Fisher SE, Vargha-Khadem F, Watkins KE, et al. Localisation of a gene implicated in a severe speech and language disorder. Nat Genet 1998;18:168–70.

[76] Vargha-Khadem F, Watkins KE, Price CJ, et al. Neural basis of an inherited speech and language disorder. Proc Natl Acad Sci U S A 1998;95:12695–700.

[77] Watkins KE, Vargha-Khadem F, Ashburner J, et al. MRI analysis of an inherited speech and language disorder: structural brain abnormalities. Brain 2002;125:465–78.

[78] Price CJ, McCrory E. Functional brain imaging studies of skilled reading and developmental dyslexia. In: Snowling MJ, Hulme C, editors. The science of reading: a handbook. Oxford: Blackwell Publishing; 2005. p. 473–96.

[79] Demonet JF, Taylor MJ, Chaix Y. Developmental dyslexia. Lancet 2004;363:1451–60.

[80] Shaywitz SE, Shaywitz BA, Fulbright RK, et al. Neural systems for compensation and persistence: young adult outcome of childhood reading disability. Biol Psychiatry 2003;54: 25–33.

[81] Hugdahl K, Gundersen H, Brekke C, et al. FMRI brain activation in a Finnish family with specific language impairment compared with a normal control group. J Speech Lang Hear Res 2004;47:162–72.

[82] Weismer SE, Plante E, Jones M, et al. A functional magnetic resonance imaging investigation of verbal working memory in adolescents with specific language impairment. J Speech Lang Hear Res 2005;48:405–25.

[83] Pennington BF, Olson RK. Genetics of dyslexia. In: Snowling M, Hulme C, editors. The science of reading: a handbook. Oxford (UK): Blackwell Publishing; 2005. p. 453–72.

[84] Fisher SE, DeFries JC. Developmental dyslexia: genetic dissection of a complex cognitive trait. Nat Rev Neurosci 2002;3:767–80.

[85] Petryshen TL, Kaplan BJ, Fu Liu M, et al. Evidence for a susceptibility locus on chromosome 6q influencing phonological coding dyslexia. Am J Med Genet 2001;105:507–17.

[86] Hsiung GY, Kaplan BJ, Petryshen TL, et al. A dyslexia susceptibility locus (DYX7) linked to dopamine D4 receptor (DRD4) region on chromosome 11p15.5. Am J Med Genet B Neuropsychiatr Genet 2004;125:112–9.

[87] Fisher SE, Francks C. Genes, cognition and dyslexia: learning to read the genome. Trends Cogn Sci 2006;10:250–7.

[88] McGrath LM, Smith SD, Pennington BF. Breakthroughs in the search for dyslexia candidate genes. Trends Mol Med 2006;12:333–41.

[89] Taipale M, Kaminen N, Nopola-Hemmi J, et al. A candidate gene for developmental dyslexia encodes a nuclear tetratricopeptide repeat domain protein dynamically regulated in brain. Proc Natl Acad Sci U S A 2003;100:11553–8.

[90] Scerri TS, Fisher SE, Francks C, et al. Putative functional alleles of DYX1C1 are not associated with dyslexia susceptibility in a large sample of sibling pairs form the UK. J Med Genet 2004;41(11):853–7.

[91] Marino C, Giorda R, Luisa Lorusso M, et al. A family-based association study does not support DYX1C1 on 15q21.3 as a candidate gene in developmental dyslexia. Eur J Hum Genet 2005;13:491–9.

[92] Bellini G, Bravaccio C, Calamoneri F, et al. No evidence for association between dyslexia and DYX1C1 functional variants in a group of children and adolescents from southern Italy. J Mol Neurosci 2005;27:311–4.

[93] Meng H, Hager K, Held M, et al. TDT-association analysis of EKN1 and dyslexia in a Colorado twin cohort. Hum Genet 2005;118:87–90.

[94] Cope NA, Hill G, van den Bree M, et al. No support for association between dyslexia susceptibility 1 candidate 1 and developmental dyslexia. Mol Psychiatry 2005;10:237–8.

[95] Wigg KG, Couto JM, Feng Y, et al. Support for EKN1 as the susceptibility locus for dyslexia on 15q21. Mol Psychiatry 2004;9:1111–21.

[96] Hannula-Jouppi K, Kaminen-Ahola N, Taipale M, et al. The axon guidance receptor gene ROBO1 is a candidate gene for developmental dyslexia. PLoS Genet 2005;1:467–74.

[97] Meng H, Smith SD, Hager K, et al. DCDC2 is associated with reading disability and modulates neuronal development in the brain. Proc Natl Acad Sci U S A 2005;102:17053–8.

[98] Cope N, Harold D, Hill G, et al. Strong evidence that KIAA0319 on chromosome 6p is a susceptibility gene for developmental dyslexia. Am J Hum Genet 2005;76:581–91.

[99] Schumacher J, Anthoni H, Dahdouh F, et al. Strong genetic evidence of DCDC2 as a susceptibility gene for dyslexia. Am J Hum Genet 2006;78:52–62.

[100] Paracchini S, Thomas A, Castro S, et al. The chromosome 6p22 haplotype associated with dyslexia reduces the expression of KIAA0319, a novel gene involved in neuronal migration. Hum Mol Genet 2006;15:1659–66.

[101] Wang Y, Paramasivan M, Thomas A, et al. Dyx1c1 functions in neuronal migration in developing neocortex. Neurosci 2006;143:515–22.

[102] Andrews W, Liapi A, Plachez C, et al. Robo1 regulates the development of major axon tracts and interneuron migration in the forebrain. Development 2006;133:2243–52.

[103] Galaburda AM, LoTurco J, Ramus F, et al. From genes to behavior in developmental dyslexia. Nat Neurosci 2006;9(10):1213–7.

[104] Hurst JA, Baraitser M, Auger E, et al. An extended family with a dominantly inherited speech disorder. Dev Med Child Neurol 1990;32:347–55.

[105] Lai CS, Fisher SE, Hurst JA, et al. A forkhead-domain gene is mutated in a severe speech and language disorder. Nature 2001;413:519–23.

[106] Lewis BA, Cox NJ, Byard PJ. Segregation analysis of speech and language disorders. Behav Genet 1993;23:291–7.

[107] Bartlett CW, Flax JF, Logue MW, et al. A major susceptibility locus for specific language impairment is located on 13q21. Am J Hum Genet 2002;71:45–55.

[108] SLI-Consortium. A genomewide scan identifies two novel loci involved in specific language impairment. Am J Hum Genet 2002;70:384–98.

[109] SLI-Consortium. Highly significant linkage to the SLI1 locus in an expanded sample of individuals affected by specific language impairment. Am J Hum Genet 2004;74:1225–38.

[110] MacDermot KD, Bonora E, Sykes N, et al. Identification of FOXP2 truncation as a novel cause of developmental speech and language deficits. Am J Hum Genet 2005;76:1074–80.

[111] Smith SD, Pennington BF, Boada R, et al. Linkage of speech sound disorder to reading disability loci. J Child Psychol Psychiatry 2005;46:1057–66.

[112] Stein CM, Schick JH, Gerry Taylor H, et al. Pleiotropic effects of a chromosome 3 locus on speech-sound disorder and reading. Am J Hum Genet 2004;74:283–97.

[113] Miscimarra L, Stein C, Millard C, et al. Further evidence of pietropy influencing speech and language: analysis of the DYX6 region. Hum Hered 2007;63:47–58.

[114] Stein CM, Millard C, Kluge A, et al. Speech sound disorder influenced by a locus in 15q14 region. Behav Genet 2006;95:153–93.

[115] McGrath LM, Pennington, BF, Willcutt EG, et al. Gene × environment interactions in speech sound disorder. Dev Psychopathol, in press.

[116] Bronfenbrenner U, Ceci SJ. Nature-nurture reconceptualized in developmental perspective: a bioecological model. Psychol Rev 1994;101:568–86.

[117] Caspi A, McClay J, Moffitt TE, et al. Role of genotype in the cycle of violence in maltreated children. Science 2002;297:851–4.

[118] Caspi A, Sugden K, Moffitt TE, et al. Influence of life stress on depression: moderation by a polymorphism in the 5-HTT gene. Science 2003;301:386–9.

PEDIATRIC CLINICS
OF NORTH AMERICA

Pediatr Clin N Am 54 (2007) 563–583

Brain Abnormalities in Language Disorders and in Autism

Martha R. Herbert, MD, PhD[a,b,*], Tal Kenet, PhD[a]

[a]Department of Neurology, Massachusetts General Hospital, MGH/Martinos,
CNY-149-6012, 149 13th Street, Charlestown, MA 02129, USA
[b]TRANSCEND Research Program, Center for Child and Adolescent Development,
Cambridge Health Alliance, Harvard Medical School, 101 Station Landing,
Medford, MA 02155, USA

Autism is defined by a triad of deficits in the domains of behavior, social skills, and communication. The communication deficits are often, although not always, accompanied by a deficit in language. Language deficits in autism can range from very mild to very severe, and involve a complete lack of language in the more extreme cases, with many such individuals remaining nonverbal throughout life. In the milder cases, in which children with autism do develop language, it is delayed in onset and remains impaired relative to peers over time. The classes of language impairments observed in children who have autism are largely heterogeneous and can span any or all of semantics, syntax, morphology, phonology, and pragmatics. Additionally, the receptive expressive impairments may be impacted to different extents. Despite the heterogeneity of language disorders in autism, the impairments in those who do speak suggest parallels to other language disorders, particularly specific language impairment (SLI). SLI is defined as language impairment in the setting of normal intelligence and in the absence of physical, anatomic, environmental, or social factors that may account for it. SLI is also heterogeneous in its presentation, but often children who have SLI exhibit many of the same language difficulties as children who have autism [1–4]. The exact nature of the similarities and differences in language abilities between autism and SLI has been addressed extensively in those articles and therefore is not reviewed here. In addition to shared language impairments between the two populations, there is also an increased rate of

This work was supported by NS48455 from NINDS, the Cure Autism Now Foundation, and the Bernard Fund for Autism Research.
* Corresponding author. Department of Neurology, Massachusetts General Hospital, MGH/Martinose, CNY-149-6012, 149 13th Street, Charlestown, MA 02129.
E-mail address: mherbert1@partners.org (M.R. Herbert).

non-autistic language impairment in relatives of people who have autism [5–9] and of autism in siblings of children who have SLI [10], suggesting some common genetic risk factors for SLI and autism.

The evidence for shared underlying mechanisms between autism and SLI is not limited to language skills and genetics. This article focuses on some of the known brain functional and anatomic overlaps (and differences) between the two disorders. Brain-based structural and functional investigations are among the many domains in which there is a growing body of evidence suggesting that some common neural substrates may underlie autism and SLI. When these conditions have been studied separately, which historically has been the case for the most part, they have been studied differently regarding regions or functions and measures and methods. In studies that consider them together and use similar or identical methodologies it becomes more possible to assess for commonalities and for differences. To date, there are few published studies in which SLI and autism groups are directly compared. Although there are also few studies of SLI using brain imaging techniques, there are many studies investigating the brain correlates of dyslexia. Individuals who have dyslexia are often language impaired, and it has been argued that the distinction between dyslexia and SLI may be more quantitative than qualitative [3], or alternatively, that the two disorders are distinct but have a strong potential for comorbidity [11]. This apparent overlap between the two disorders suggests that here too there may be shared underlying neural substrates between dyslexia and SLI. Because of this, it is conceivable that some of the findings in dyslexia may also be pertinent to SLI and to autism. It is particularly interesting to study the dyslexia literature in this regard, because, like in autism, many non–language-specific (both anatomic and functional) abnormalities have been documented in the population, some of which overlap partially or strongly with deficits described in autism, as discussed later in this article.

The findings of abnormalities in non–language-specific domains are of particular interest, because they highlight a basic methodologic challenge that faces the study of the brain in language disorders. That is, do we focus our study of brain abnormalities on the areas known to be associated with language functions? Or do we investigate the brain more broadly, to contextualize language-area abnormalities and to seek other abnormalities that may also, or even instead, be primary in driving the deficits? It has been argued that from the vantage point of brain development the latter is more appropriate, given that developmental mechanisms start as domain-general rather than domain-specific [12], and the dysregulation of such mechanisms that presumably underlies developmental disorders, including autism and SLI, is therefore likely to have widespread impacts.

Because both autism and SLI involve language deficits, language-associated brain structure and function has been a focus of study in both conditions. This methodologic question has been answered differently in these two disorders. The deficits beyond language in autism, which are central to the disorder's definition, have driven autism brain researchers to study many areas, structures, and functions of the brain, particularly given the lack of prior clarity about the brain localization of the pertinent non-language functions, whereas the more subtle non-language abnormalities in SLI have not motivated a similarly broad investigative range in SLI brain research. Still, as research progresses we have accumulated ample evidence from electroencephalogram (EEG), magnetoencephalogram (MEG), functional MRI, and anatomic MRI of brain abnormalities outside of language-associated structures and functions, and such evidence is accumulating also in SLI and other disorders associated with language impairments, especially dyslexia. Because there is a relative lack of comparable functional brain imaging studies between SLI (or dyslexia) and autism in the language domain, and because this issue has been addressed elsewhere in relative detail [1,2,4,13,14], this article focuses on other functional studies in which comparisons can be made, which are all in the domains of sensory perception of simple stimuli. This early sensory perception domain is of particular interest given some of the more recent hypotheses raised in the literature, that sensory perception may be degraded because of a low intrinsic cortical signal-to-noise ratio [15], which may in turn lead to degraded internal representations of the external world, including language. If these current trends in research lead to further understanding of common mechanisms and underlying pathophysiology, such understanding could very well help us develop more effectively targeted treatments and interventions, either medically addressing features of the underlying pathophysiology or using training methods to address features of perturbed sensory processing.

Macroanatomy

Asymmetry

The populational predominance of leftward lateralization of language functions has made the study of asymmetry attractive in autism and SLI, because it is known that there is a higher frequency of ambidextrousness, left-handedness, or right hemisphere language dominance in individuals who have language disorders and autism. This question has been pursued in imaging studies of autism and SLI subjects, but it has been addressed differently in the two groups. We address large-scale, local, and comprehensive asymmetry assessments.

In autism and SLI studies, large-scale asymmetries have been a modest but persistent theme in the literature and were among the first differences from controls to be documented. CT scans were found to reveal "unfavorable" anatomic asymmetries in autism [16]. The same authors also found reversed asymmetry by CT in subjects who had speech delay [17]. A large-scale rightward shift in autism and a childhood speech disorder (dysphasia) has been previously reported in two functional studies. Resting regional cerebral blood flow asymmetry was shifted from predominantly left to predominantly right in an autistic [18] and a dysphasic group [19]. This ratio shift had a different origin in each group. In the autism group this reversal of right-to-left ratio was driven by regional cerebral blood flow that was no different from controls on the right but diminished on the left, whereas in the dysphasia group the left regional cerebral blood flow was largely unchanged and the right was increased. There thus appears to be less overall cerebral blood flow in the autistic sample and more in the dysphasic one.

Local asymmetries

MRI studies in SLI have largely focused on gyri and sulci in the inferior frontal, perisylvian, and posterior sylvian regions, but the measures used have differed among studies. Perisylvian abnormalities have been found in several SLI cohorts. A neuropathologic study found atypical planum temporale (PT) asymmetry and a dysplastic gyrus on the inferior left frontal cortex [20]. Imaging studies have included reports of altered PT asymmetry [21], but also PT asymmetry that was unchanged from controls in length measures [22] or volume measures [23], although one of these studies reported no size difference [22], whereas the other reported that the PT was bilaterally smaller in proportion to smaller forebrain size [23].

Loss or reversal of perisylvian asymmetry was found in six of eight SLI subjects [21]. This finding was accompanied by widespread bilateral abnormalities in neighboring perisylvian regions; however, no one specific abnormality was present in all subjects. Atypical perisylvian asymmetries were also reported in most parents and siblings of a group of affected children [24]. Right-sided perisylvian volumes were larger in some SLI children [25], whereas in another study the left posterior perisylvian region was smaller in more than half of the SLI subjects as compared with only one of the controls [26]. A relationship between measures of facial affect skills and variation in the right supramarginal gyrus was interpreted as evidence of right hemisphere involvement in the non-language deficits in subjects who had SLI [27].

Inferior frontal abnormalities that have been reported include morphologic variants of the inferior frontal gyrus in family members of children who have SLI [28] and more common occurrence of an extra sulcus in the inferior frontal gyrus in adult subjects who have behavioral signs consistent with history of a language disorder [29]. In another study, the inferior frontal gyrus, pars triangularis, was smaller on the left in children who had SLI [22].

In autism research there have been no studies until recently comparable to SLI investigations of perisylvian gyri and sulci. Although a recent study showed widespread variation in sulcal anatomy, its measures were not comparable to those used in prior SLI studies [30]. Rojas and colleagues [31] reported a significant reduction of left PT volume but no change in the right hemisphere; Heschl's gyrus was also measured but no differences were found, and the region was leftwardly asymmetric in both groups. A voxel-based morphometry study found decreased volume in the left inferior temporal gyrus [32]. In a study of high-functioning boys who had autism, our own group has reported a volume asymmetry reversal in inferior frontal cortex with accompanying asymmetry differences in planum temporale and posterior temporal fusiform gyrus compared with controls [33]; we also found a leftward planum temporale asymmetry different from controls in SLI not present in our controls [34]. A later study replicating this method of investigation in a new cohort found reversed inferior frontal asymmetry in SLI and in subjects who had autism and language impairments, but not in typically developing controls or in subjects who had autism and normal language scores [14].

Widely distributed asymmetry changes

In general there are few comprehensive studies of regional asymmetries throughout the brain, and this is also true in the autism and SLI brain research literature. Our own group reported a whole-brain investigation of volumetric asymmetries, however, examining anatomic structures and regions in a nested hierarchy in a comparison of high-functioning boys who had autism (in whom we had previously reported reversed inferior frontal asymmetry), boys who had developmental language disorder, and age-matched controls. No group showed asymmetry at the level of total hemispheric volumes; lobar asymmetry was manifested only in the controls and only regarding a leftward asymmetry in the frontal lobes. In cerebral cortex gyral regions, however, there was a marked increase in rightward asymmetry in both autism and SLI that was widely distributed in the brain in a highly similar distribution in both groups, and that was especially prominent in higher-order associational areas. The striking similarity in asymmetry alterations in these groups suggests that (1) asymmetries may be significant far beyond language regions, (2) the alterations may be systematic rather than random, and (3) asymmetry alterations in language-associated regions may be a subcomponent of a much more pervasive pattern of anatomic perturbation. This set of similarities also raises the question of whether there may be other widespread changes in anatomic and functional domains. Moreover, the greater degree of asymmetry alterations in higher-order associational areas, whose development is more experience expectant, suggests a potentially important role for epigenetic factors in the development of asymmetry. A recent MEG study of a modest number of late childhood and adolescent subjects showing an increase in rightward asymmetry in autism and of leftward asymmetry in controls with increasing age supports this inference [35].

Other brain regional differences

Thalamus/diencephalon

Cortical coordination, relevant to complex functions such as language, involves the thalamus. Thalamic volume reduction and loss of correlation with total brain volume was found in high-functioning young adults who had autism [36], whereas an early MRI study also found a trend toward reduced thalamic volume, but only on the right [37]. In school-aged boys who had autism and SLI Jernigan and colleagues [26] reported a reduction in right diencephalic volume. In our own studies we measured diencephalon, which included thalamus and hypothalamus. Diencephalon was significantly larger in our high-functioning school-age boys who had autism but not in those who had SLI, compared with controls (and the autistic volume was no different from controls after adjustment for total brain volume) [38,39].

Physical coordination abnormalities have been documented in SLI [40] and autism [41,42], bringing to mind possible basal ganglia and cerebellar correlates. Basal ganglia volume differences have been found in autism, with some studies showing smaller volume [37], some no difference [43], and some larger volume [38,44]. In SLI studies, the intergenerational KE family cohort, whose affected members manifest a severe inherited articulatory speech and language disorder [45,46], bilaterally reduced caudate volume was revealed by voxel-based morphometry and subsequent more detailed volumetric measures. The severe oromotor deficits in this family are not typical in SLI subjects more broadly, however. In other volumetric measures, one study found a trend toward smaller right caudate but no differences in left caudate or lenticulate (globus-pallidus and putamen) in either hemisphere [26].

There is a large body of literature on cerebellar volume alterations in autism that has been substantially reviewed elsewhere. Although the cerebellum may be important in language disorders, given the increasing appreciation of its role in cognitive processes [47] there are almost no studies of the cerebellum in SLI. There have been a few studies of cerebellum in dyslexia, however, with findings including loss of cerebellar asymmetry [48], smaller right anterior cerebellar lobe [49], and altered right anterior cerebellar lobe symmetry [50], with converging support from measurements of metabolic [51] and neuropathologic [52] abnormalities. These abnormal cerebellar findings have been associated with the motor abnormalities found in these children, in the form of a cerebellar deficit hypothesis [53,54]. In this formulation, the non–language-related deficits found in many children who have dyslexia are characterized as one manifestation of a general impairment in the ability to perform skills automatically, with automatization of skills being mediated by the cerebellum.

Widely distributed and nonuniform volumetric differences

Brain volume

A tendency toward larger brains (ie, increase in brain size, head size, or brain weight) is the most replicated anatomic finding in autism. About 20% have head circumference measures above the 90th percentile, and most are above average [55–57]. The volume increase occurs postnatally, with meta-analysis of cross-sectional studies of differently aged cohorts suggesting a rapid increase during the first 2 years with a sharp subsequent falloff in growth rate compared with controls [58]. Hazlett and colleagues [59] measured brain volumes in a cohort at risk for autism through age 2 years and found enlargement of cerebral gray and white matter but not of cerebellum. Aylward and colleagues [60] measured head circumference and brain volume and found that both measures were larger in children less than 12 years old who had autism, whereas only head circumference was larger in older individuals who had autism, suggesting an early rapid brain growth with the volume initially achieved not being maintained through the life course.

There have been few measures of total brain volume in SLI. Our own research has yielded the first reported documentation of increased brain volume in SLI [39], a dimension that has largely gone unmeasured in language-oriented neuroanatomic studies. In these data, mean total brain volumes were measured to be larger for both autism and SLI than for controls, and these volume measures were also larger in autism than in SLI. One prior study of head circumference in autism and semantic pragmatic disorder found more non-autistic language-disordered children than controls with macrocephalic head circumference [61], whereas the only MRI volumetric study to report brain volume of which we are aware found forebrain volume 7% smaller in SLI than in controls [62]. Large brains do not seem to be found in other disorders, such as bipolar disorder and schizophrenia [63].

Cerebral cortex

Widespread changes in cortical surface anatomy were discerned in a study assessing position of prominent sulci [30]. A voxel-based morphometry study of young adults who had autism showed decreased gray matter in the right paracingulate sulcus, left inferior frontal gyrus, and left occipito-temporal junction, and increased gray matter in the left periamygdaloid cortex, left middle temporal gyrus, and right inferior temporal gyrus [32]. A voxel-based morphometric study of SLI in a single family (the KE family) with a severe dominantly inherited global SLI showed less gray matter in right and left sensorimotor cortex and right and left inferior temporal gyrus, with more gray matter in the left inferior frontal gyrus, left anterior insular cortex, left and right precentral gyrus, and medial occipitoparietal cortex [46].

White matter and brain enlargement

It seems that the increased brain volume in autism is largely driven by an increase in white matter. In a study of 2- to 16-year-olds, white matter enlargement was found in 2- to 3-year-old autistic children, whereas 12- to 16-year-old autistic children had less white matter than controls [64]. In the younger children, moreover, although the autistic group had 18%

more cerebral white matter, in the cerebellum the white matter volume increase was 38%.

For SLI, the one report of gray and white matter volumes in children does not include any age-matched controls [65]. Among the adults in that study, however, the language-impaired group had a decreased gray-to-white ratio compared with adult controls, with more white matter and less gray matter. This difference was attributed to generalized atrophy, although it is unclear why atrophy would be associated with or result in increased white matter volume.

In our own study population, white matter is the only region that is absolutely and proportionally increased in either our autism or our SLI samples. White matter is 15% larger in boys who have autism than in controls [38]. In SLI it is 8% larger in boys and 18% larger in girls [39]. Because of the difficulty in finding high-functioning girls to enroll in imaging studies and the great difficulties involved in scanning low-functioning subjects who have autism, little is known about the volumetrics of autism in girls, although a national effort to pool the small samples from multiple studies is underway. White matter constitutes a disproportionate 66% of the total brain volume increase in autism and 88% of the brain volume increase in SLI in our cohorts.

In the white matter itself, radiate white matter (ie, subjacent to the cortex) is significantly enlarged, whereas deep sagittal, bridging, and descending tracts are not. Radiate white matter is affected in all lobes in autism but the parietal is spared in SLI; however, in both disorders the prefrontal lobe is affected most prominently, being 36% larger in autism and 26% larger in SLI than controls. Areas myelinating later or for longer showed greater enlargement [66]. Making sense of the contribution of large brain volume to observed functional impairments can be attempted either through looking at areas where brain volume overlaps with relevant distributed neural systems or through considering the network impacts of disruption of long-tract connectivity [57]; further research using functional and structural modalities will investigate which modeling approach is the best fit, but selectively considering only brain regions associated with behavioral or linguistic phenotypic features when the changes are much more widespread seems problematic.

Corpus callosum

The corpus callosum has been of interest in SLI and autism, because interhemispheric transfer is relevant to various hypotheses about the functional abnormalities, including asymmetry, in both disorders. In autism, two studies have found the corpus callosum to be smaller, mostly posteriorly [67,68]. A further study, in subjects who had mentally retardation and autism, found volume reduction mostly in the body of the corpus callosum [69]. Yet another study found volume reduction in the anterior of the corpus [70]. In SLI, one study found no difference in midsagittal callosal area [62], whereas another measured the corpus to be thicker in children who had familial dysphasia/dyslexia [71]. In our own samples [66], we found no difference in either SLI or autism in the midsagittal area of the corpus callosum, either as a whole or in any of the specific subregions delineated according to the method of Witelson [72]; however, the lack of volume increase occurred in the setting of larger brain and white matter volume, which ought to have lead to a larger corpus callosum because corpus callosum normally covaries to the 2/3 power of brain volume [73].

Implications of macroanatomic findings

At the level of regional measures there is substantial variability between many of the studies, some clearly attributable to methodology or age differences and some not easily explained and perhaps representing differences between cohorts in these undoubtedly heterogeneous disorders. The field of view shifts, however, with the finding of large brains not only in autism but also in SLI. These findings highlight a previously unrecognized void in SLI brain studies, which have hitherto been focused overwhelmingly on language-associated parts of the brain. We are observing differences in the scaling or volumetric proportionality of the brain that may reflect pervasively altered ratios of convergence and divergence in processing systems [74]. At present, the functional impact of such an anatomic change is not easily explained [57], although the accompanying sharp increases in rightward cortical asymmetry in both groups may hint at some aspect of this impact. But these commonalities between disorders suggest a pathophysiology that is not only shared but also widely distributed in its impact across functional domains. It also suggests that the underlying pathophysiology at the level of molecular, cellular, and tissue mechanisms may target physical features that overlap only partially and perhaps even coincidentally with the regional distributions of neural systems as they relate to neurocognitive processing [75]. This physical targeting could account for the widespread physical changes in autistic and SLI brains that we have recounted, and it could also represent physical concomitants of functional disruptions that could involve a widely distributed reduction in the signal-to-noise ratio that we began to discuss in our introduction. Our review of sensory perception in these disorders that further pursues this line of thought follows from the need to investigate potential commonalities at basic levels of functioning that may be associated with such widespread structural changes.

Functional abnormalities

Sensory perception deficits in autism

Autism has been linked with impairments in simple sensory perception early in the hierarchy of cortical processing, in the visual [76–81] and auditory [82–88] domains, and to some extent also in the somatosensory domain

[89], although those data are so far mostly anecdotal. To date, the correlation between these sensory impairments and the behavioral characteristics of autism remains unknown. More specifically, the extent to which some of the higher-order deficits associated with autism could be downstream consequences of low-level sensory perception abnormalities is still an open question. The investigation of sensory perception deficits in autism encompasses an additional dimension; some similar deficits have been described also in children who have language impairments, further underscoring the importance of understanding the nature of the neurobiologic mechanisms that may be shared between autism and SLI. This section of the article focuses on three classes of low-level sensory perception that have been studied in autism and in either SLI or dyslexia, both of which are on the spectrum of language disorders, that have been stipulated to play a role in the core deficits of those disorders: (1) visual processing of nonbiologic (random dots) motion; (2) visual processing as a function of signal-to-noise ratio; and (3) auditory processing of tone stimuli.

Motion perception

A common paradigm used to study the perception of motion uses randomly placed moving dots, referred to as random dots kinematogram (RDK). The percentage of dots moving in the same direction is defined as coherence; (ie, if 40% of the dots are moving to the right and another 60% are moving randomly, the stimulus has 40% coherence). The goal is to find the threshold, or the minimal coherence level, for detection of the direction of motion of the coherent dots. This measure is defined as the motion coherence threshold (MCT). The paradigm was first pioneered in the 1980s on experiments in primates [90], and was shown to be highly effective in activating middle temporal cortex (MT, also known as V5 in humans). Furthermore, it was shown that MT activation was directly correlated with the direction of movement of the dots and with behavioral reports [91]. This paradigm has since been explored in many different populations, including dyslexia and autism.

In dyslexia, the RDK paradigm became popular because it taps into the magnocellular or dorsal stream hypothesis of dyslexia, which states, in brief, that individuals who have dyslexia process rapid visual signals poorly, a function attributed to the magnocellular (dorsal) stream [92]. There is a general agreement between groups that individuals who have dyslexia, both adults and children, are impaired on this task and on average have higher MCT, indicating a deficit on this paradigm. It is now generally accepted that this failure is not sufficient to conclude the existence of a particular dorsal stream deficit, however, and the issue remains actively debated. Although there are no studies investigating RDK thresholds in children who have language impairments, it has been shown that a significant proportion of children who have dyslexia also have language impairments [3,11], making it highly likely that similar deficits will also be observed in SLI populations.

In autism, the RDK paradigm has been explored behaviorally using psychophysics techniques by several groups [76,80,93], all of whom found that individuals who have autism have significantly higher detection thresholds (ie, higher MCT) than controls. Interpretations of the common finding, however, have varied. Some interpret the higher MCT in autism as evidence for a dorsal stream deficit that has been hypothesized also in dyslexia [76,93] In support of this claim, Spencer and colleagues also tested performance on a parallel task using static lines oriented concentrically, instead of dots. The coherence (or level of noise) was defined by the number of lines oriented randomly as opposed to concentrically. On this latter task, which tests sensitivity to form, children who have autism were similar to controls, and hence the group concluded that the deficits are confined to the dorsal stream. In a parallel exploration, Pellicano and colleagues [80] compared the performance of the autism group on the RDK task to their performance on a flicker contrast task. Their hypothesis was that the former targets *later* dorsal stream functions, whereas the latter targets *earlier* levels of the cortical dorsal stream. They further compared the performance on each of these tasks to the child's performance on a task that tested the child's level of central coherence. Although they found no differences between the groups in the flicker contrast task, they found that children who had autism were impaired on RDK and central coherence tasks, the latter being in agreement with the weak central coherence (WCC) hypothesis of autism [94–96]. They used the children's intact performance on the parallel flicker contrast task to rule out attentional and other confounding effects, and concluded that it is the later levels of the dorsal stream (V5) that must be affected, whereas earlier levels of the dorsal stream (V1/V2) remain intact. Pellicano and colleagues [97] raised the possibility, later explored in greater detail in a review by Dakin and Frith [79], that WCC is correlated with impairment on the RDK task. Specifically, the hypothesis put forth by Dakin and Frith is that it is the *integration* across the moving dots that is impaired in autism. This hypothesis creates a natural link between this relatively lower-order phenomenon of random dot motion and the perception of biologic motion, which is known to be impaired in autism [79,98] and is usually considered a higher-order social cognition capacity. One prediction of this hypothesis is that in autism, early response patterns are identical to those of typically developing children and differ only at later times of the response, indicating feedback interference from higher areas. Such a prediction is in agreement with Schulte-Korne and colleagues [99] but has yet to be tested.

The noise exclusion hypothesis

In their study of the perception of visual motion in autism, Bertone and colleagues [78] used a different approach from the one presented above. The group differentiated between luminance-defined (first order) motion, and texture-defined (second order) motion. They found that individuals who have autism have thresholds of detection that are similar to controls for first-order motion stimuli but are impaired on detecting second-order motion stimuli. The authors interpret their results as a deficit in the perception of *complex* stimuli, rather than a deficit along the magnocellular stream. This hypothesis is in line with at least two other studies of sensory perception in dyslexia. The first of these is by Talcott and colleagues [100], who used the RDK stimulus described above to examine motion perception in dyslexia. They found that if more dots are added to the RDK, children who have dyslexia improve and at very high dot density levels actually become indistinguishable from controls in their performance. Talcott and colleagues suggest this positive effect of increasing the motion energy could imply that individuals who have dyslexia have inherently *lower signal-to-noise ratios*. They conclude that poor signal-to-noise perception may play a part in dyslexia. Another study that generated a lot of attention in the field of dyslexia is by the group of Sperling and colleagues [101], who found that the thresholds of children who had dyslexia for detection of monochromatic gratings in noise varied not with whether the gratings were optimized for the parvo- (high spatial frequency) or magno- (low spatial frequency) streams; instead, thresholds varied only with the level of noise in which the gratings were embedded. They concluded that individuals who have dyslexia have a deficit in noise exclusion rather than in any particular stream of processing. Their finding has an additional angle that makes it particularly pertinent to autism despite the differences between autism and dyslexia; Sperling and colleagues find that it is the individuals who have dyslexia but are also *language impaired* who are most affected by the noise. Although they did not examine children who had language impairment but not dyslexia, their finding makes it highly likely that it may be that language impairments play a major role in driving the deficit in noise exclusion, rather than just the dyslexia. The above studies hint toward poor signal-to-noise ratios, or degraded internal cortical representations of stimuli, in language-impaired, dyslexic, and autistic populations in the visual domain.

Auditory processing abnormalities

There is ample evidence that children who have autism process the sounds of speech [35,88,102–104] and voices [104–106] differently from typically developing children. There is an ongoing debate regarding whether or not this impairment stems from a more primary sensory perception deficit in the processing of auditory information, however. There are many studies showing that, in fact, children who have autism also have abnormal processing of nonspeech sounds, such as tones, which occurs early in the auditory cortical hierarchy relative to language processing. Those include abnormal mismatch response in the frequency domain [88,107–109], gap detection in the temporal domain [110], and abnormal magnitude perception/neuronal response in the intensity domain [83,111]. Of these, one study did compare children who had autism directly with language-impaired individuals [110], and the two populations were found to have similar deficits in the processing of tones presented in a rapid sequence. In parallel to the studies of the perception of tone stimuli in autism there is also literature examining the processing of tone stimuli in SLI. Although at least one group found no difference in tone mismatch response around the frequency axis [112], other studies show a behavioral deficit in children who have SLI that is specific to frequency discrimination [113], which is also manifested using electrophysiologic markers. Abnormalities in the structure of N1 have been described in both dyslexia and SLI [114] and in autism [87]. All of the above evidence indicates that deficits in the processing of language may begin at cortical levels that precede language areas, through impairments in rapid processing, abnormal N1 that in turn may result in a degraded signal passed forward to language areas, and abnormal change detection, all of which are critical for language perception. In parallel to this evidence, at least in autism, some groups do find normal evoked response potentials (ERPs) for non-speech stimuli, and abnormal ERPs only in response to speech stimuli in autism [103,106]. The reasons for there discrepancy between findings remain to be explored and resolved.

Implications of functional abnormalities

Although there is strong support of sensory perception abnormalities in autism and SLI, it is not known whether associations exist between these lower-order sensory perception processes in which these abnormalities have been documented and higher-order processes that reflect on social perception (eg, biologic motion, theory of mind, and language). Although both populations (autism and SLI/dyslexia) seem to share several classes of sensory perception abnormalities, abnormalities in social function have only been documented in autism to date, suggesting that perhaps social cognition and social perception could follow a pathway that does not dependent entirely on early sensory perception. Additionally, it has recently been shown that theory of mind is independent of language ability [115], further suggesting that social cognition is indeed a strong differentiator between these two disorders. To further understand the nature of the overlap between autism and SLI, one would have to turn to studies that interrelate sensory and social perception.

The functional findings described above are also important to view in the context of diagnosis, cause, treatment, and prognosis. Language disorders and autism spectrum disorders are defined behaviorally, and are usually only identified between roughly 18 months (for autism) and early school years (for dyslexia). Delineating a set of functional measures that could determine risk independently of and possibly before the emergence of diagnosis-specific behaviors would increase the likelihood of early detection, which in turn could facilitate early intervention and therefore improve prognosis. Such measures could potentially be easily obtained using an EEG cap and a set of passive or otherwise simple stimuli, which have the advantage of requiring minimal cooperation from the infant or toddler. Additionally, functional measures that do not rely on behavioral response may provide a fresh means for parsing subtypes within each disorder, and thus potentially allow us to gain insight into the etiology and pathophysiology of each of these disorders, for which the current grouping into a single disorder confounds research. Furthermore, such measures could open the door for individualized or better-tailored therapies that correlate with the severity of each specific set of functional abnormalities (eg, visual, auditory, motion) identified in each individual.

Neuropathology and pathophysiologic considerations

Moving down from macroanatomy to tissue rather than up to function in the biologic hierarchy leads to neuropathology and cellular and molecular pathophysiology. There is a modest amount of neuropathologic literature in autism, almost none in SLI, and some in dyslexia. Findings in dyslexia have included ectopia, altered asymmetries, abnormal minicolumns [116], and abnormalities in the magnocellular system. Animal models developed to pursue some of these findings show an association between ectopia and lesion-induced microgyria with impaired temporal processing [117,118], an interesting correlation of a local physical abnormality with a more pervasive functional problem. In autism, neuropathologic findings include heavy brains, abnormal cell-packing density in the limbic system, and widely distributed patchy cortical abnormalities [119,120], along with nicotinic and GABAergic receptor abnormalities [121,122]. More recently neuroinflammation (with abnormal innate but not adaptive immunity in the affected brains) and signs of oxidative stress have been identified in every brain studied in a set of autistic postmortem samples ranging from ages 3 to 44 [123–125]. This finding, along with observations of changes in cellular size in older compared with younger brains, suggests a different class of pathophysiology, apparently ongoing through the life course [119], that may be associated with neurochemical changes that could degrade the signal-to-noise ratio and thus lead to some of the functional consequences described above, although this functional association has not been pursued in published studies. Although there are no studies investigating this phenomenon in SLI, a debate about the role of the immune system is ongoing in autism and language disorders [126–130].

Summary

We have reviewed local and widespread anatomic changes in SLI and autism, and substantial but not complete similarities between the two disorders, and we have reported suggestive sensory processing abnormalities across domains. The findings we have reported go substantially beyond the structural and functional domains that would be uniquely altered if these disorders were based on genes or pathophysiologic processes that specifically targeted the neural substrates of language processing. They lend broad support to models of widespread processing deficits deriving from early domain-general dysregulations of brain development that impair language but also impair many other domains, although not to equal degrees across the board. The non-language impairments in SLI could be a consequence of these widespread processing deficits, and impairments in autism (such as anxiety, abnormal sensory thresholds, and sleep disorders) that are outside of the three defining domains of impairments could also be part of the same overall picture. Abnormal immune system findings in at least some individuals who have autism and SLI (and in some family members in both disorders) may be pertinent to underlying molecular and cellular pathophysiology, although there is no way at present to know the proportion of individuals who have either autism or SLI to whom this is relevant.

Sensory impairments early in the processing hierarchy and pervasive brain changes, such as brain enlargement, may conceivably be early signs of impairment that could be detected before the onset of the specific phenotypic features diagnostic of autism and SLI. This observation raises the prospect of developing biomarkers for early identification, and such biomarkers may also be pertinent to designing early interventions and predicting which individuals might benefit most from such interventions.

Whatever the underlying biology, these widely distributed anatomic and cross-modal sensory findings, and suggestions of overlapping genetic and pathophysiologic processes that might drive such brain structural and functional changes, lead us to seek greater specificity regarding what is driving the anatomic changes and what is driving the alterations in sensory-perceptual domains. To address such questions, we need a multilevel research program. We need to identify subgroups and parse heterogeneity within diagnostic groups, because we do not currently know whether the variations in findings between studies represent methodologic differences or intrinsic differences between individuals and cohorts. We need more studies with comparable methods to enable intergroup comparison. We also need to pay attention more systematically to the physical features in these brains, using methodologies such as magnetic resonance spectroscopy to characterize metabolites and diffusion tensor imaging and other cutting-edge in vivo methods to characterize tissue, in association with high temporal resolution measures from EEG and MEG to assess whether and how timing and other functional alterations are correlated with tissue changes. We need to integrate genetic and pathophysiologic studies to gain insight into whether there are similar or different underlying mechanisms for language impairment in some or all subgroups of each diagnostic category. Finally, we need to apply these insights to treatment development. The identification of vulnerabilities or disease processes in some individuals could lead to medical treatments for those subgroups, whereas the characterization of timing abnormalities could help shape novel neural systems rehabilitation approaches. Our review supports our claim that the rubric of language disorders provides at the same time an organizing focus and a challenge to explain the non-language features. This tension should continue to provoke fruitful investigations and will help improve the quality of life of affected individuals.

References

[1] Bishop DV. Autism and specific language impairment: categorical distinction or continuum? Novartis Found Symp 2003;251:213–26 [discussion: 226–34, 281–97].

[2] Bishop DV, Norbury CF. Exploring the borderlands of autistic disorder and specific language impairment: a study using standardised diagnostic instruments. J Child Psychol Psychiatry 2002;43(7):917–29.

[3] Bishop DV, Snowling MJ. Developmental dyslexia and specific language impairment: same or different? Psychol Bull 2004;130(6):858–86.

[4] Kjelgaard MM, Tager-Flusberg H. An investigation of language impairment in autism: implications for genetic subgroups. Lang Cogn Process 2001;16(2/3):287–308.

[5] Fombonne E, Bolton P, Prior J, et al. A family study of autism: cognitive patterns and levels in parents and siblings. J Child Psychol Psychiatry 1997;38(6):667–83.

[6] Piven J, Palmer P, Jacobi D, et al. Broader autism phenotype: evidence from a family history study of multiple-incidence autism families. Am J Psychiatry 1997;154(2):185–90.

[7] Piven J, Palmer P. Cognitive deficits in parents from multiple-incidence autism families. J Child Psychol Psychiatry 1997;38(8):1011–21.

[8] Piven J, Palmer P, Landa R, et al. Personality and language characteristics in parents from multiple-incidence autism families. Am J Med Genet 1997;74(4):398–411.

[9] Bolton PF, Veltman MW, Weisblatt E, et al. Chromosome 15q11-13 abnormalities and other medical conditions in individuals with autism spectrum disorders. Psychiatr Genet 2004;14(3):131–7.

[10] Tomblin JB, Hafeman LL, O'Brien M. Autism and autism risk in siblings of children with specific language impairment. Int J Lang Commun Disord 2003;38(3):235–50.

[11] Catts HW, Adlof SM, Hogan TP, et al. Are specific language impairment and dyslexia distinct disorders? J Speech Lang Hear Res 2005;48(6):1378–96.

[12] Karmiloff-Smith A. The tortuous route from genes to behavior: a neuroconstructivist approach. Cogn Affect Behav Neurosci 2006;6(1):9–17.

[13] Botting N, Conti-Ramsden G. Autism, primary pragmatic difficulties, and specific language impairment: can we distinguish them using psycholinguistic markers? Dev Med Child Neurol 2003;45(8):515–24.

[14] De Fosse L, Hodge SM, Makris N, et al. Language-association cortex asymmetry in autism and specific language impairment. Ann Neurol 2004;56(6):757–66.

[15] Rubenstein JL, Merzenich MM. Model of autism: increased ratio of excitation/inhibition in key neural systems. Genes Brain Behav 2003;2(5):255–67.

[16] Hier DB, LeMay M, Rosenberger PB. Autism and unfavorable left-right asymmetries of the brain. J Autism Dev Disord 1979;9(2):153–9.

[17] Rosenberger PB, Hier DB. Cerebral asymmetry and verbal intellectual deficits. Ann Neurol 1980;8(3):300–4.

[18] Chiron C, Leboyer M, Leon F, et al. SPECT of the brain in childhood autism: evidence for a lack of normal hemispheric asymmetry. Dev Med Child Neurol 1995;37(10):849–60.

[19] Chiron C, Pinton F, Masure MC, et al. Hemispheric specialization using SPECT and stimulation tasks in children with dysphasia and dystrophia. Dev Med Child Neurol 1999;41(8): 512–20.

[20] Cohen M, Campbell R, Yaghmai F. Neuropathological abnormalities in developmental dysphasia. Ann Neurol 1989;25(6):567–70.

[21] Plante E, Swisher L, Vance R, et al. MRI findings in boys with specific language impairment. Brain Lang 1991;41(1):52–66.

[22] Gauger LM, Lombardino LJ, Leonard CM. Brain morphology in children with specific language impairment. J Speech Lang Hear Res 1997;40(6):1272–84.

[23] Preis S, Jancke L, Schittler P. Normal intrasylvian anatomical asymmetry in children with developmental language disorder. Neuropsychologia 1998;36(9):849–55.

[24] Plante E. MRI findings in the parents and siblings of specifically language-impaired boys. Brain Lang 1991;41(1):67–80.

[25] Filipek P, Richelme C, Kennedy D, et al. Morphometric analysis of the brain in developmental language disorders and autism [abstract]. Ann Neurol 1992;32:475.

[26] Jernigan TL, Hesselink JR, Sowell E, et al. Cerebral structure on magnetic resonance imaging in language- and learning-impaired children. Arch Neurol 1991;48(5):539–45.

[27] Plante E, Boliek C, Mahendra N, et al. Right hemisphere contribution to developmental language disorder: neuroanatomical and behavioral evidence. J Commun Disord 2001; 34(5):415–36.

[28] Jackson T, Plante E. Gyral morphology in the posterior Sylvian region in families affected by developmental language disorder. Neuropsychol Rev 1996;6(2):81–94.

[29] Clark MM, Plante E. Morphology of the inferior frontal gyrus in developmentally language-disordered adults. Brain Lang 1998;61(2):288–303.

[30] Levitt JG, Blanton RE, Smalley S, et al. Cortical sulcal maps in autism. Cereb Cortex 2003; 13(7):728–35.

[31] Rojas DC, Bawn SD, Benkers TL, et al. Smaller left hemisphere planum temporale in adults with autistic disorder. Neurosci Lett 2002;328(3):237–40.

[32] Abell F, Krams M, Ashburner J, et al. The neuroanatomy of autism: a voxel-based whole brain analysis of structural scans. Neuroreport 1999;10(8):1647–51.

[33] Herbert MR, Harris GJ, Adrien KT, et al. Abnormal asymmetry in language association cortex in autism. Ann Neurol 2002;52(5):588–96.

[34] Herbert MR, Ziegler DA, Makris N, et al. Increased cerebral white matter and brain volume in children with developmental language disorder. Ann Neurol 2002;52(3):S114–5.

[35] Flagg EJ, Cardy JE, Roberts W, et al. Language lateralization development in children with autism: insights from the late field magnetoencephalogram. Neurosci Lett 2005;386(2): 82–7.

[36] Tsatsanis KD, Rourke BP, Klin A, et al. Reduced thalamic volume in high-functioning individuals with autism. Biol Psychiatry 2003;53(2):121–9.

[37] Gaffney GR, Kuperman S, Tsai LY, et al. Forebrain structure in infantile autism. J Am Acad Child Adolesc Psychiatry 1989;28(4):534–7.

[38] Herbert MR, Ziegler DA, Deutsch CK, et al. Dissociations of cerebral cortex, subcortical and cerebral white matter volumes in autistic boys. Brain 2003;126(Pt 5):1182–92.

[39] Herbert MR, Ziegler DA, Deutsch CK, et al. Brain asymmetries in autism and developmental language disorder: a nested whole-brain anaylsis. Brain 2005;128(2):213–26.

[40] Hill EL. Non-specific nature of specific language impairment: a review of the literature with regard to concomitant motor impairments. Int J Lang Commun Disord 2001;36(2): 149–71.

[41] Minshew NJ, Sung K, Jones BL, et al. Underdevelopment of the postural control system in autism. Neurology 2004;63(11):2056–61.

[42] Teitelbaum P, Teitelbaum O, Nye J, et al. Movement analysis in infancy may be useful for early diagnosis of autism. Proc Natl Acad Sci U S A 1998;95(23):13982–7.

[43] Hardan AY, Kilpatrick M, Keshavan MS, et al. Motor performance and anatomic magnetic resonance imaging (MRI) of the basal ganglia in autism. J Child Neurol 2003;18(5): 317–24.

[44] Sears LL, Vest C, Mohamed S, et al. An MRI study of the basal ganglia in autism. Prog Neuropsychopharmacol Biol Psychiatry 1999;23(4):613–24.

[45] Vargha-Khadem F, Watkins KE, Price CJ, et al. Neural basis of an inherited speech and language disorder. Proc Natl Acad Sci U S A 1998;95(21):12695–700.

[46] Watkins KE, Vargha-Khadem F, Ashburner J, et al. MRI analysis of an inherited speech and language disorder: structural brain abnormalities. Brain 2002;125(Pt 3):465–78.

[47] Schmahmann JD, Caplan D. Cognition, emotion and the cerebellum. Brain 2006;129(Pt 2): 290–2.

[48] Rae C, Harasty JA, Dzendrowskyj TE, et al. Cerebellar morphology in developmental dyslexia. Neuropsychologia 2002;40(8):1285–92.

[49] Eckert MA, Leonard CM, Richards TL, et al. Anatomical correlates of dyslexia: frontal and cerebellar findings. Brain 2003;126(Pt 2):482–94.

[50] Leonard CM, Lombardino LJ, Walsh K, et al. Anatomical risk factors that distinguish dyslexia from SLI predict reading skill in normal children. J Commun Disord 2002;35(6): 501–31.

[51] Rae C, Lee MA, Dixon RM, et al. Metabolic abnormalities in developmental dyslexia detected by 1H magnetic resonance spectroscopy. Lancet 1998;351(9119):1849–52.

[52] Finch AJ, Nicolson RI, Fawcett AJ. Evidence for a neuroanatomical difference within the olivo-cerebellar pathway of adults with dyslexia. Cortex 2002;38(4):529–39.

[53] Zeffiro T, Eden G. The cerebellum and dyslexia: perpetrator or innocent bystander? Trends Neurosci 2001;24(9):512–3.

[54] Ivry RB, Justus TC. A neural instantiation of the motor theory of speech perception. Trends Neurosci 2001;24(9):513–5.

[55] Rapin I, editor. Preschool children with inadequate communication: developmental language disorder, autism, low IQ. London: Mac Keith Press; 1996. [Clinics in Developmental Medicine; 139].

[56] Bauman ML, Kemper TL. Histoanatomic observations of the brain in early infantile autism. Neurology 1985;35:866–74.

[57] Herbert MR. Large brains in autism: the challenge of pervasive abnormality. Neuroscientist 2005;11(5):417–40.

[58] Redcay E, Courchesne E. When is the brain enlarged in autism? A meta-analysis of all brain size reports. Biol Psychiatry 2005;58(1):1–9.

[59] Hazlett HC, Poe M, Gerig G, et al. Magnetic resonance imaging and head circumference study of brain size in autism: birth through age 2 years. Arch Gen Psychiatry 2005; 62(12):1366–76.

[60] Aylward EH, Minshew NJ, Field K, et al. Effects of age on brain volume and head circumference in autism. Neurology 2002;59(2):175–83.

[61] Woodhouse W, Bailey A, Rutter M, et al. Head circumference in autism and other pervasive developmental disorders. J Child Psychol Psychiatry 1996;37(6):665–71.

[62] Preis S, Steinmetz H, Knorr U, et al. Corpus callosum size in children with developmental language disorder. Brain Res Cogn Brain Res 2000;10(1–2):37–44.

[63] Ward KE, Friedman L, Wise A, et al. Meta-analysis of brain and cranial size in schizophrenia. Schizophr Res 1996;22(3):197–213.

[64] Courchesne E, Karns CM, Davis HR, et al. Unusual brain growth patterns in early life in patients with autistic disorder: an MRI study. Neurology 2001;57(2):245–54.

[65] Kabani NJ, MacDonald D, Evans A, et al. Neuroanatomical correlates of familial language impairment: a preliminary report. J Neurolinguistics. vol. 10(2–3), 1997. p. 203–14. [Elsevier Science Ltd, England 1997]

[66] Herbert MR, Ziegler DA, Makris N, et al. Localization of white matter volume increase in autism and developmental language disorder. Ann Neurol 2004;55(4):530–40.

[67] Egaas B, Courchesne E, Saitoh O. Reduced size of corpus callosum in autism. Arch Neurol 1995;52(8):794–801.
[68] Piven J, Bailey J, Ranson BJ, et al. An MRI study of the corpus callosum in autism. Am J Psychiatry 1997;154(8):1051–6.
[69] Manes F, Piven J, Vrancic D, et al. An MRI study of the corpus callosum and cerebellum in mentally retarded autistic individuals. J Neuropsychiatry Clin Neurosci 1999;11(4):470–4.
[70] Hardan AY, Minshew NJ, Keshavan MS. Corpus callosum size in autism. Neurology 2000; 55(7):1033–6.
[71] Njiokiktjien C, de Sonneville L, Vaal J. Callosal size in children with learning disabilities. Behav Brain Res 1994;64(1–2):213–8.
[72] Witelson SF. Hand and sex differences in the isthmus and genu of the corpus callosum: a postmortem morphological study. Brain 1989;112:799–835.
[73] Jancke L, Staiger JF, Schlaug G, et al. The relationship between corpus callosum size and forebrain volume. Cereb Cortex 1997;7(1):48–56.
[74] Ziegler DA, Herbert MR, Hodge SM, et al. Disproportionate linear scaling of cerebral white to gray matter in boys with autism and developmental language disorder. Society for Neuroscience. Program No. 124.7. 2002.
[75] Herbert MR, Ziegler DA. Volumetric neuroimaging and low-dose early-life exposures: loose coupling of pathogenesis-brain-behavior links. Neurotoxicology 2005;26(4):565–72.
[76] Milne E, Swettenham J, Hansen P, et al. High motion coherence thresholds in children with autism. J Child Psychol Psychiatry 2002;43(2):255–63.
[77] Bertone A, Mottron L, Jelenic P, et al. Motion perception in autism: a "complex" issue. J Cogn Neurosci 2003;15(2):218–25.
[78] Bertone A, Mottron L, Jelenic P, et al. Enhanced and diminished visuo-spatial information processing in autism depends on stimulus complexity. Brain 2005;128(Pt 10):2430–41.
[79] Dakin S, Frith U. Vagaries of visual perception in autism. Neuron 2005;48(3):497–507.
[80] Pellicano E, Gibson L, Maybery M, et al. Abnormal global processing along the dorsal visual pathway in autism: a possible mechanism for weak visuospatial coherence? Neuropsychologia 2005;43(7):1044–53.
[81] Davis RA, Bockbrader MA, Murphy RR, et al. Subjective perceptual distortions and visual dysfunction in children with autism. J Autism Dev Disord 2006;36(2):199–210.
[82] Gomot M, Giard MH, Adrien JL, et al. Hypersensitivity to acoustic change in children with autism: electrophysiological evidence of left frontal cortex dysfunctioning. Psychophysiology 2002;39(5):577–84.
[83] Bruneau N, Bonnet-Brilhault F, Gomot M, et al. Cortical auditory processing and communication in children with autism: electrophysiological/behavioral relations. Int J Psychophysiol 2003;51(1):17–25.
[84] Gomot M, Bernard FA, Davis MH, et al. Change detection in children with autism: an auditory event-related fMRI study. Neuroimage 2006;29(2):475–84.
[85] Gage NM, Siegel B, Roberts TP. Cortical auditory system maturational abnormalities in children with autism disorder: an MEG investigation. Brain Res Dev Brain Res 2003; 144(2):201–9.
[86] Gage NM, Siegel B, Callen M, et al. Cortical sound processing in children with autism disorder: an MEG investigation. Neuroreport 2003;14(16):2047–51.
[87] Bomba MD, Pang EW. Cortical auditory evoked potentials in autism: a review. Int J Psychophysiol 2004;53(3):161–9.
[88] Oram Cardy JE, Flagg EJ, Roberts W, et al. Delayed mismatch field for speech and non-speech sounds in children with autism. Neuroreport 2005;16(5):521–5.
[89] Edelson SM, Edelson MG, Kerr DC, et al. Behavioral and physiological effects of deep pressure on children with autism: a pilot study evaluating the efficacy of Grandin's Hug Machine. Am J Occup Ther 1999;53(2):145–52.
[90] Newsome WT, Pare EB. A selective impairment of motion perception following lesions of the middle temporal visual area (MT). J Neurosci 1988;8(6):2201–11.

[91] Salzman CD, Newsome WT. Neural mechanisms for forming a perceptual decision. Science 1994;264(5156):231–7.

[92] Habib M. The neurological basis of developmental dyslexia: an overview and working hypothesis. Brain 2000;123(Pt 12):2373–99.

[93] Spencer J, O'Brien J, Riggs K, et al. Motion processing in autism: evidence for a dorsal stream deficiency. Neuroreport 2000;11(12):2765–7.

[94] Frith U, Happe F. Autism: beyond "theory of mind". Cognition 1994;50(1–3):115–32.

[95] Castelli F, Frith C, Happe F, et al. Autism, Asperger syndrome and brain mechanisms for the attribution of mental states to animated shapes. Brain 2002;125(Pt 8):1839–49.

[96] Happe F, Frith U. The weak coherence account: detail-focused cognitive style in autism spectrum disorders. J Autism Dev Disord 2006;36(1):5–25.

[97] Pellicano E, Maybery M, Durkin K. Central coherence in typically developing preschoolers: does it cohere and does it relate to mindreading and executive control? J Child Psychol Psychiatry 2005;46(5):533–47.

[98] Blake R, Turner LM, Smoski MJ, et al. Visual recognition of biological motion is impaired in children with autism. Psychol Sci 2003;14(2):151–7.

[99] Schulte-Korne G, Bartling J, Deimel W, et al. Visual evoked potential elicited by coherently moving dots in dyslexic children. Neurosci Lett 2004;357(3):207–10.

[100] Talcott JB, Hansen PC, Assoku EL, et al. Visual motion sensitivity in dyslexia: evidence for temporal and energy integration deficits. Neuropsychologia 2000;38(7):935–43.

[101] Sperling AJ, Lu Z-L, Manis FR, et al. Deficits in perceptual noise exclusion in developmental dyslexia. Nat Neurosci 2005;8(7):862–3.

[102] Kasai K, Hashimoto O, Kawakubo Y, et al. Delayed automatic detection of change in speech sounds in adults with autism: a magnetoencephalographic study. Clin Neurophysiol 2005;116(7):1655–64.

[103] Kuhl PK, Coffey-Corina S, Padden D, et al. Links between social and linguistic processing of speech in preschool children with autism: behavioral and electrophysiological measures. Dev Sci 2005;8(1):F1–12.

[104] Lepisto T, Kujala T, Vanhala R, et al. The discrimination of and orienting to speech and non-speech sounds in children with autism. Brain Res 2005;1066(1–2):147–57.

[105] Gervais H, Belin P, Boddaert N, et al. Abnormal cortical voice processing in autism. Nat Neurosci 2004;7(8):801–2.

[106] Ceponiene R, Lepisto T, Shestakova A, et al. Speech-sound-selective auditory impairment in children with autism: they can perceive but do not attend. Proc Natl Acad Sci U S A 2003; 100(9):5567–72.

[107] Seri S, Cerquiglini A, Pisani F, et al. Autism in tuberous sclerosis: evoked potential evidence for a deficit in auditory sensory processing. Clin Neurophysiol 1999;110(10):1825–30.

[108] Ferri R, Elia M, Agarwal N, et al. The mismatch negativity and the P3a components of the auditory event-related potentials in autistic low-functioning subjects. Clin Neurophysiol 2003;114(9):1671–80.

[109] Tecchio F, Benassi F, Zappasodi F, et al. Auditory sensory processing in autism: a magnetoencephalographic study. Biol Psychiatry 2003;54(6):647–54.

[110] Oram Cardy JE, Flagg EJ, Roberts W, et al. Magnetoencephalography identifies rapid temporal processing deficit in autism and language impairment. Neuroreport 2005;16(4): 329–32.

[111] Khalfa S, Bruneau N, Roge B, et al. Increased perception of loudness in autism. Hear Res 2004;198(1–2):87–92.

[112] Uwer R, Albrecht R, von Suchodoletz W. Automatic processing of tones and speech stimuli in children with specific language impairment. Dev Med Child Neurol 2002; 44(8):527–32.

[113] McArthur GM, Bishop DV. Speech and non-speech processing in people with specific language impairment: a behavioural and electrophysiological study. Brain Lang 2005;94(3): 260–73.

[114] Leppanen PH, Lyytinen H. Auditory event-related potentials in the study of developmental language-related disorders. Audiol Neurootol 1997;2(5):308–40.

[115] Colle L, Baron-Cohen S, Hill J. Do children with autism have a theory of mind? A non-verbal test of autism vs. specific language impairment. J Autism Dev Disord 2006.

[116] Casanova MF, Buxhoeveden DP, Cohen M, et al. Minicolumnar pathology in dyslexia. Ann Neurol 2002;52(1):108–10.

[117] Fitch RH, Tallal P, Brown CP, et al. Induced microgyria and auditory temporal processing in rats: a model for language impairment? Cereb Cortex 1994;4(3):260–70.

[118] Frenkel M, Sherman GF, Bashan KA, et al. Neocortical ectopias are associated with attenuated neurophysiological responses to rapidly changing auditory stimuli. Neuroreport 2000;11(3):575–9.

[119] Bauman ML, Kemper TL. Neuroanatomic observations of the brain in autism: a review and future directions. Int J Dev Neurosci 2005;23(2–3):183–7.

[120] Bailey A, Luthert P, Dean A, et al. A clinicopathological study of autism. Brain 1998;121 (Pt 5):889–905.

[121] Perry EK, Lee ML, Martin-Ruiz CM, et al. Cholinergic activity in autism: abnormalities in the cerebral cortex and basal forebrain. Am J Psychiatry 2001;158(7):1058–66.

[122] Blatt GJ. GABAergic cerebellar system in autism: a neuropathological and developmental perspective. Int Rev Neurobiol 2005;71:167–78.

[123] Vargas DL, Nascimbene C, Krishnan C, et al. Neuroglial activation and neuroinflammation in the brain of patients with autism. Ann Neurol 2005;57(1):67–81.

[124] Vargas DL, Bandaru V, Zerrate MC, et al. Oxidative stress in brain tissues from autistic patients: increased concentration of isoprostanes. IMFAR 2006. Poster PS2.6. Montreal (Canada), June 2006.

[125] Perry G, Nunomura A, Harris P, et al. Is autism a disease of oxidative stress? Presented at the Oxidative Stress in Autism Symposium, New York State Institute for Basic Research in Developmental Disabilities. Staten Island (NY), June 16, 2005. p. 15.

[126] Ashwood P, Van de Water J. A review of autism and the immune response. Clin Dev Immunol 2004;11(2):165–74.

[127] Ashwood P, Van de Water J. Is autism an autoimmune disease? Autoimmun Rev 2004; 3(7–8):557–62.

[128] Hornig M, Lipkin WI. Infectious and immune factors in the pathogenesis of neurodevelopmental disorders: epidemiology, hypotheses, and animal models. Ment Retard Dev Disabil Res Rev 2001;7(3):200–10.

[129] Dalton P, Deacon R, Blamire A, et al. Maternal neuronal antibodies associated with autism and a language disorder. Ann Neurol 2003;53(4):533–7.

[130] Benasich AA. Impaired processing of brief, rapidly presented auditory cues in infants with a family history of autoimmune disorder. Dev Neuropsychol 2002;22(1):351–72.

PEDIATRIC CLINICS
OF NORTH AMERICA

ELSEVIER
SAUNDERS

Pediatr Clin N Am 54 (2007) 585–607

Using the Language Characteristics of Clinical Populations to Understand Normal Language Development

Heidi M. Feldman, MD, PhD

*Department of Pediatrics, Stanford University School of Medicine,
750 Welch Road Suite 315, Palo Alto, CA 94304, USA*

The speech and language characteristics of children who have hearing loss and neurologic conditions shed light on the requirements of language learning under normal circumstances. Adverse outcomes of moderate to profound hearing loss are mitigated by amplification or cochlear implantation. The age of treatment is associated with outcome, demonstrating the important role of auditory input in infancy for organizing speech perception and language neural systems. Early insertion of tympanostomy tubes for otitis media with effusion and associated minimal to mild hearing loss reduces the duration of effusion but does not improve outcomes in comparison to delayed or no tympanostomy tube insertion. These observations suggest that variable, intermittent, mild hearing loss is not sufficient to disrupt language development in otherwise healthy children. Low socioeconomic status is associated with greater delays in speech and language than is otitis media with effusion, demonstrating the importance of the quantity and quality of early verbal input. Early focal brain injury to areas of the brain associated with language processing in adulthood is often associated with good outcomes in terms of speech, language, and cognition. Functional imaging studies show that uninjured areas of the right hemisphere, not associated with language under normal circumstances, become active during language tasks in children who have early left-hemisphere injury. These observations indicate that the neural substrate for language is not specialized at birth but evolves in the process of language learning. Children who have acquired diffuse traumatic brain injury have less favorable outcomes than children who have focal injuries, demonstrating the limits of plasticity. Together these observational studies demonstrate that the verbal environment and process of language learning affect brain organization and language skills.

E-mail address: hfeldman@stanford.edu

The overall purpose of this article is to describe the speech and language abilities of children who have selected clinical conditions, not only to characterize the outcomes of those conditions, but also to understand fundamental requirements for language learning in typically developing children. This developmental cognitive neuroscience analysis conceptualizes the clinical conditions as naturalistic experimental manipulations, selectively altering factors in the language-learning situation that could not otherwise be ethically manipulated in a research study. By describing the outcomes in such cases, researchers can evaluate the impact of those factors on the developmental course. This article uses several clinical conditions to explore the role of the verbal language environment and of specialized neural organization on speech and language development. Table 1 summarizes the broad, general requirements for normal speech and language development and the clinical conditions and disorders that may interfere with them in the normal developmental processes.

We know generally that children learn speech and language from their environment. After all, American children learn English, Brazilian children learn Portuguese, and Filipino children learn Tagalog. Children gain access to the verbal language environment through the auditory system. Studies of children who have hearing loss can be conceptualized as natural experiments regarding the role of audition and verbal input on language development. Studies of children who have profound sensorineural hearing loss demonstrate the impact of severe permanent hearing loss on speech and language. Studies of children who have profound hearing loss treated with cochlear implantation, or moderate to severe hearing loss treated with amplification at different ages, can be used to demonstrate the impact of permanent hearing loss at varying levels and for varying durations on the developmental processes. Studies of children who have conductive hearing loss from otitis media can be used to evaluate the impact of intermittent minimal to mild hearing loss on speech and language. This article contrasts the language development of children who have hearing loss with that of children of low socioeconomic status, who often experience an impoverished language environment despite adequate hearing.

Table 1
General requirements for language learning that may be disrupted by clinical conditions

Requirements for language learning	Access to verbal language environment	Specialized neural organization
Problems that compromise language development	Limited access to input	Abnormal neural structures or functions
Clinical conditions	Hearing impairment; impoverished verbal input, low SES	Focal brain injury, traumatic brain injury; epileptiform disorders

We also know that the human brain is required for language learning. Dolphins and nonhuman primates have sophisticated communication systems and yet fail to develop symbolic systems as complex as human language. The left hemisphere of the human has a specialized role in language functioning in adults. Aphasia, the severe disruption of language functions after brain damage is associated with left-hemisphere injury in 95% of adult cases. Studies of children who have focal neural injuries to the left-hemisphere language areas of the brain can demonstrate whether this neural specialization is innate or acquired through exposure to the verbal environment and process of language learning. Functional imaging studies can be used to determine the neural organization of language in children who have damage to classic language areas and nonetheless learn to speak. This article contrasts the development of children who have focal injury to that of children who have traumatic brain injury and Landau-Kleffner syndrome, an acquired aphasia associated with abnormal epileptiform discharge, to demonstrate the differences in outcomes after focal versus diffuse neural injuries.

From the review of these clinical examples, the resiliency of language development under many conditions of hearing loss and neural injury becomes apparent. Early exposure to a rich and varied verbal environment is essential for organizing the speech and language systems. The specialized neural organization of language is not firmly established before language development but rather develops through the process of language development. This developmental specialization provides mechanisms for plasticity in the face of clinical conditions that might otherwise derail the developmental process. Severe untreated hearing loss and bilateral neural injuries show the vulnerability of language development in extreme cases. These findings have important implications for clinical practice and public policy.

Hearing impairment

Definitions and conceptual basis

Access to the verbal language environment requires the auditory system. Hearing loss can compromise that access. Speech sounds generally fall within the frequency ranges of 500 to 4000 Hz. Conversational speech is typically composed of sounds with an energy level that ranges from 50 to 60 decibels. Some speech sounds, including vowels and consonants/m and b/ are composed of low frequency energy. Some speech sounds, including consonants and especially/$s, f,$ and th/, are composed of high frequency energy. Some speech sounds, such as the/th/in the word *thin* are weak or low energy, and some are intense, such as the vowel/aw/or high energy.

The degree of hearing loss is described as mild, moderate, severe, and profound. The specific thresholds for these levels of hearing loss vary across texts [1]. Children who have profound hearing loss have hearing thresholds greater than 80 decibels. They are not able to hear much of routine conversational language, even with the benefit of hearing aids. Children who have severe hearing loss have thresholds of 60 to 80 decibels. They rely on hearing aids and may still have difficulty detecting and interpreting speech sounds. Children who have moderate hearing loss have thresholds of 40 to 60 decibels; they have considerable difficulty hearing speech without the use of a hearing aid. Children who have mild hearing loss have thresholds of 20 to 40 decibels; they may have difficulty deciphering speech, particularly in noisy environments.

Amplification is the mainstay of treatment for hearing loss. Children who have severe to profound hearing loss who do not benefit from amplification may be candidates for cochlear implantation. Outcomes in terms of speech and language as a function of the degree of hearing loss and the type and age of treatment are important clinical issues. How outcomes vary as a function of impaired access to an adequate verbal environment versus unimpaired access to an impoverished environment is also relevant to theoretic accounts of language development as well as clinical and public policy.

Severe to profound hearing loss

Findings

Children who have severe to profound hearing loss generally have marked limitations in speech and verbal language [2]. Because they cannot learn oral language readily from environmental exposure, they require extensive training in all available visual and auditory information (including lips, facial expression, and environmental cues) to perceive and interpret verbal language. They also require intensive education in speech production. Despite special education, these children are highly unlikely to develop strong speech perception and production skills. One reason for persistent difficulties is that lip reading alone without the benefit of auditory information cannot be used to discriminate among many sounds. For example, the distinction between /b/ and /p/ or /d/ and /t/ cannot be appreciated from the appearance of the mouth. Another reason is that auditory input and feedback remains important for normal speech production. Many children who have severe and profound hearing loss and are educated only in aural/oral methods eventually create a manual communication system for use with family and friends [3,4] or switch to sign language when they enter schools for the deaf [5].

In the current era, many children who have severe to profound hearing loss who do not benefit from amplification are candidates for cochlear implantation. Cochlear implants are prosthetic devices that bypass the abnormal cochlea, stimulate the auditory nerve, and allow the individual to sense sound. The implants consist of a microphone to amplify environmental sounds, a speech processor, a transmitter, and a set of electrodes surgically placed on the cochlea to stimulate the auditory nerve.

Children treated with cochlear implantation have better speech, verbal language, and reading skills than children who have comparable losses who do not have the implants [6–8]. They are more likely to attend mainstream schools. However, their outcomes are variable. Children who have the best outcomes develop abilities to understand speech and converse competently. Children who have fair outcomes use the information from the implant to improve their skills at speech reading or to increase their awareness of environmental sounds [9]. As a group, children who have cochlear implants do not do as well as children who have normal hearing in terms of speech perception, speech production, and academic skills [6,10]. However, their ultimate skills are comparable to children who have moderate to severe hearing loss, treated with conventional hearing aids [11]. The younger the age of the child is at the time of implantation, the better the outcome [12–14].

Implications

Persistent differences in the outcomes of children who have early amplification and cochlear implants compared with the outcomes of children who have normal hearing [10] implicate the importance of a rich auditory signal and/or exposure to verbal language in early infancy for learning speech and language. At the present time, it is difficult to differentiate which of these factors is more important in the development of speech and language. However, as the technology of cochlear implants improves, creating a more complex auditory signal, and as the age of implantation decreases to 1 year or younger, the data may become available to distinguish which of these factors is most relevant.

The variability in outcomes not accounted for by the age of implantation emphasizes that multiple factors are associated with speech and language development beyond the acuity of hearing. We know from other studies that genetic factors, for example, are associated with specific language impairment, a condition in which language skills are significantly impaired in comparison to intelligence and other skills [15–17]. In addition, language skills correlate with general intellectual abilities. However, these factors may be difficult to modify in the effort to improve outcomes for speech and language skills among children who have severe to profound hearing loss. Other factors, such as educational strategies, exposure to manual language or total communication, and family adaptation, should be aggressively studied to determine their importance in the development of speech and language in children who have severe hearing loss to improve outcomes.

Mild to moderate sensorineural hearing loss

Findings

The number of studies on the outcomes of mild to moderate sensorineural hearing loss is surprising limited [18]. A population study of 86

Australian school-aged children who had mild to profound hearing loss found that the children who had hearing loss had lower scores on language and academic testing in comparison to children who had normal hearing. In addition, they had more behavior problems than the comparison group. Total language and receptive language scores on formal testing were proportional to the degree of hearing loss; children who had mild hearing loss achieved mean scores of 94.8 and 87.5 on total language and receptive vocabulary, respectively [2]. Adaptive behavior, behavior problems, and academic skills were unrelated to the degree of hearing loss. In another study, a detailed analysis of speech and language skills in a group of British children who had mild to moderate sensorineural hearing loss found that approximately half of the children had a phonologic impairment, with reduced phonologic short-term memory, discrimination, and phonologic awareness in comparison to children who had normal hearing of the same chronologic age. However, there were no differences between groups on vocabulary, sentence recall, sentence compression, or literacy [19]. This study demonstrates that broad language and academic skills may be preserved in the context of a speech disorder associated with mild to moderate hearing loss.

In the past, many children who had mild to moderate hearing loss were not identified until they reached 2 to 3 years old and were already behind in language development. They missed considerable auditory input during their first few months of life when the auditory system is organizing the speech perception apparatus around the specific sounds of the native language [20]. In the era of Universal Newborn Hearing Screening, children who have congenital mild to moderate sensorineural hearing losses should be identified in the first 3 months of life and provided amplification by 6 months of age. Studies will be able to show whether restoring hearing in the first 6 months of life eradicates the linguistic and academic disadvantage of mild to moderate hearing loss. Unfortunately, randomized clinical trials of the outcomes of universal newborn hearing screening in comparison to other detection methods were not accomplished before the change in public policies mandating screening [21]. In the era before universal screening, amplification by 6 months of age for children who had mild to profound hearing loss was associated with improvements in cognitive, receptive, and expressive language outcomes in comparison to amplification older than 6 months of age [22]. In the early amplification cohort, the degree of hearing loss did not influence outcomes. A more recent study compared children identified immediately before and after the introduction of universal screening in regions of the United Kingdom [23]. This study compared the individual children's speech and language scores to their nonverbal abilities using z-scores for various tests. The results showed language benefits for confirmation of hearing loss before 9 months of age. Improvements were demonstrated in receptive language scores after introduction of universal screening, but not in expressive language or speech [23].

Implications

More research is needed on children who have mild to moderate sensori-neural hearing loss. In the era of universal newborn hearing screening, it should be much easier than in the past to identify cohorts of children who have received early and effective amplification. The outcomes under these ideal circumstances will contribute to understanding the role of auditory input on speech and language. Of course, it may be difficult to identify control groups of any size whose congenital hearing loss was not identified until later ages. However, we may be able to determine whether amplification by 2 to 3 months of age offers greater benefit than amplification at 6 months.

Otitis media with effusion

Findings

After the common cold, otitis media is the most commonly diagnosed illness in children. Approximately one half to two thirds of healthy children who have otitis media with effusion but no other developmental disorder or high-risk status experience hearing loss. On average their auditory threshold increases by 10 to 15 decibels [24]. Though approximately 5% of children have hearing loss of 40 to 50 decibels [25], the typical hearing loss is at worst mild. Otitis media occurs most frequently in the first 3 years of life, the period of most rapid language development. Because of the disruption of normal hearing in this important period of the child's life, many clinicians and researchers have been concerned that otitis media may cause long-standing disruptions in speech and language development in children who are frequently or severely affected.

A recent review of the literature found that the duration of middle ear effusion is minimally associated with later unfavorable outcomes in terms of speech, language, cognition, attention, and academic skills [25]. However, such associations do not imply a causal relationship. The duration of otitis media with effusion is associated with various adverse socioeconomic and environmental conditions, including low socioeconomic status, smoking in the household, short durations of breastfeeding, young age of the mother, and contact with many children [26]. Associations between the quality of the home or day care environment and developmental outcomes are far greater in magnitude than the associations of duration of otitis media and those same outcomes [25]. Indeed, the impact of otitis media on developmental outcomes may be mediated by the home environment.

The most convincing evidence that otitis media with effusion does not cause adverse developmental outcomes and that insertion of tympanostomy tubes does not improve developmental outcomes comes from a large randomized clinical trial in a sociodemographically diverse sample [27–29]. In this set of studies, 6350 healthy children were followed prospectively and evaluated monthly with pneumatic otoscopy and, in many cases, tympanometry to determine the duration of middle ear effusion. A subset of 429 children reached a predefined threshold of chronic persistent middle ear effusion. They were randomly assigned to undergo tympanostomy tube placement (TTP) immediately (early TTP group) or to wait up to 9 more months and to undergo the procedure only if the effusion persisted (late or no TTP group). This random assignment successfully altered the subsequent duration of middle ear effusion in the two otherwise comparable groups. The early TTP group experienced less subsequent days of effusion than the late or no TTP group. The children were then followed to 6 years of age. The studies showed that the early and late or no TTP groups had equivalent scores on tests of receptive language, auditory processing, and intelligence. They had comparable vocabulary size and syntactic complexity in the analysis of conversational samples [27–29]. They also showed no differences in terms of the number of behavior problems on both parent and teacher rating scales [27].

Implications

These 4 studies demonstrate that in otherwise healthy children the variable and minimal hearing loss associated with otitis media with effusion within the range studied does not cause unfavorable outcomes in speech or language. It is possible that adverse effects of otitis media occur at durations shorter than the threshold for randomization. However, a high proportion of children experience effusions of such durations. A more likely explanation for the findings is that the minimal to mild degree of hearing loss is not sufficient to significantly impair perception of speech sounds. When the sample of children in the randomized clinical trials were segregated on the basis of the degree of hearing loss during prolonged bouts of effusion, the results showed that children who had poorer hearing had poorer outcomes than did children who had better hearing, but that there was no advantages of early tube placement over late or no tympanostomy placement even within the small group with a 40-decibel threshold [27]. Because relieving the effusion through tympanostomy tube placement does not alter outcomes, the finding suggests that the degree of hearing loss may be associated with other factors that cause the adverse outcomes. Another reason for finding no differences between the early and late or no tympanostomy groups may relate to our emerging understanding of the processes of language development. Recent theories in cognitive neuroscience known as "connectionist models," stress that children use far more than auditory input when they are learning language. Information from the context—conversation and environmental cues—supports the child's perception, understanding, and production. Children who have minimal to mild hearing loss are most likely able to fill in any speech that they cannot readily detect from all of the other available cues [30]. A final explanation for the lack of an effect may be that the hearing loss is variable over time. All children experience considerable variability in the speech signal. They hear males and females, adults and children, loud individuals and the soft-spoken. The speech of these different groups varies in terms of frequency and energy of sounds. They may hear native speakers and immigrants with accents whose speech sounds will vary in multiple dimensions. Connectionist models suggest that variability in the sensory signal may actually aid learning of skills, such as speech and language, because neural networks are designed to extract the invariant features of targets when presented with variations [30].

The clinical implication of the findings on otitis media is that treatment with tympanostomy tubes can be deferred if the only justification is concern about possible speech or language consequences of chronic otitis media. Future research should consider children who have other risk factors for speech and language disorders, such as Down syndrome or prematurity, to develop practice guidelines for management of otitis media in those populations.

Low socioeconomic status

Findings

Many studies document that children of low socioeconomic status experience delays in the early stages of language development compared with children from middle to high socioeconomic status. In one such study, conversation analyses and formal testing were used to evaluate speech and language skills of 240 3-year-old children in relation to three levels of maternal education—less than a high school diploma, high school graduate, and college graduate [31]. Linear trends in syntactic skills, vocabulary size, and vocabulary diversity as well as receptive vocabulary were statistically significant. Only the trend for diversity of different sounds did not reach statistical significance. Whether and when these early delays should be classified as language disorders has yet to be determined. In another association study of otitis media and language outcomes, a sample of 241 children was divided up into three groups on the basis of maternal education (<high school, high school graduate, and college graduate) and three groups on the basis of duration of otitis media (<15% days, 15%–30% days, and >30% days). The difference in mean receptive vocabulary standard scores of children who had the shortest and longest durations of middle ear effusion was 5.6 points. The difference between children whose mothers with less than high school and those whose mothers graduate college was 19.9 points [32].

The quantity and nature of parental input has been associated with the size of the child's vocabulary and with the rate of syntactic learning [33–35]. Observation studies have documented up to 10 fold differences in the amount of parental input that children hear [36]. The rate of vocabulary growth in these children was strongly influenced by the sheer amount of maternal input. Children of low socioeconomic status hear far less language and far less complex language than their middle class peers [37].

It could be argued that because vocabulary must be learned from the environment, a more interesting test of the importance of the verbal environment is syntactic development. In a study of 34 children, multiple-regression analysis determined that the proportion of multiclause sentences in parent speech was the best predictor of the number of complex sentences in the child's speech, accounting for 39% of the variance. After that, socioeconomic status accounted for only an additional 5.23% of the variance [34]. Furthermore, children's syntactic knowledge can be experimentally advanced through an educational enrichment program. Children exposed to stories with a high proportion of sentences in the passive voice developed better understanding and production of the passive voice than children who heard the same story with a low proportion of passive sentences [33].

Implications

These findings on the impact of the social environment on children's development have profound clinical and public health significance. The quantity and the quality of the verbal environment affect the developmental process. It is essential to advise parents about the importance of the early language environment for their children. Moreover, training parents who have low verbal skills or output to increase their talk to children could potentially lead to profound and long-lasting improvements in the child's language development. Reach out and Read is a program that stresses the importance of reading to infants and toddlers in the context of pediatric practice. Reading to children is an excellent strategy for increasing language input to children [38,39], which may explain its success in improving receptive language abilities in one study [40]. In terms of public health, high-quality early care and education programs may be extremely useful for children whose families are unable to provide a rich verbal environment. In such settings, teachers may require special training to provide an optimal environment for language learning. Further studies are needed to determine whether other adverse conditions associated with poverty, such as chronic stress, inadequate nutrition, and exposure to violence have a direct contribution to language learning or whether the amount and type of language input serve as the mediators between environmental factors and child language learning. Efforts to improve environmental stimulation for children who have hearing loss and children of low socioeconomic status should be rigorously evaluated in future research.

Neural injuries

Conceptual background

Aphasia can be defined as the severe disruption of language function due to neurologic injury. Aphasia is associated with injuries to the left hemisphere in approximately 95% of adult cases. Slow, halting, effortful speech production with adequate language understanding is observed in association with damage to the third convolution of the frontal lobe, a region called Broca's area. Deficits in language comprehension in the presence of fluent but meaningless speech are observed in association with damage to the posterior section of the superior temporal gyrus at the temporal–parietal junction, a region called Wernicke's area. Adults who have right-hemisphere injury may show language disturbances, but they generally have fluent but disinhibited empty speech. Many new lines of research, in particular functional imaging studies, are showing that other parts of the brain participate in language functioning and that these areas also participate in other skills [41]. Nonetheless, the severe disturbances in language following damage to the left hemisphere form the basis of the conclusion that the left hemisphere is specialized for language functioning.

When do left-hemisphere neural systems become organized for language learning? Are children born with a left hemisphere that is specialized to learn language? Alternatively, does the differentiation of the two hemispheres arise through the process of development, and in particular, language learning? One strategy for answering these important theoretic questions is the study of children who have injuries to the putative language areas of the brain before the beginnings of language development. Rarely, children experience middle cerebral artery infarctions or localized periventricular hemorrhage in the pre- or perinatal periods. Some children experience a central nervous system thrombosis or an embolic event during corrective cardiac surgery in the first few months of life. If children who have such early "prelinguistic" left-hemisphere injuries learn language at considerably slower rates than children who have right-hemisphere injuries and children developing typically, then the implication would be that the left hemisphere is specialized for language functions at the time of birth, most likely on the basis of genetic mechanisms. However, if children who have left and right-hemisphere injury perform comparably and particularly if both groups learn language at rates similar to those of children developing typically, then the implication is that other regions of the cortex are capable of serving language functioning. Furthermore, it would suggest that hemispheric differentiation arises as the result of the language learning process rather than from purely genetic mechanisms. A middle ground is also possible. If children who have left-hemisphere injury are somewhat impaired in language development or functioning compared with children who have right-hemisphere injury, the results would suggest that subtle predispositions for left-hemisphere specialization are present early in life and that the specialization becomes more marked through the process of language learning.

If the left hemisphere becomes increasingly specialized over time, then the age at which a child sustained neural injury should be relevant to outcome. Younger children who have not undergone specialization should demonstrate better outcomes than older children do because their neural substrate would be committed.

Early focal brain injuries

Findings

The outcomes of children who have prelinguistic injuries are variable and related to many factors, including the presence of a seizure disorder [42]. Children who have early focal injury to either hemisphere who are free of seizures generally begin to acquire language in the toddler–preschool period and show mild to moderate delays in the acquisition of skills. A phonologic analysis of infant babbling in a small sample of children found moderate delays in both children who had left and right-hemisphere injuries [43]. Parents report delays of word learning and emergence of early syntactic abilities on psychometrically sound survey instruments [44–46]. Longitudinal observational studies that collected conversational samples of children with their parents approximately quarterly in the toddler–preschool era confirmed these results [47,48]. In addition, using the longitudinal design it was possible not only to describe the children at any given age, but also to calculate the rate of development over time [47,48]. In terms of both vocabulary learning and syntactic skills, the children who had prelinguistic injuries functioned at normal to low normal levels for age and that their rate of development paralleled that of children developing typically.

The differences in language skills of children who have left compared with children who have right-hemisphere injury are at most minor and more pronounced in the early phases of language development. Two descriptive studies using parent report data, one regarding the acquisition of English and the other Italian, found that in early development the toddlers who had left-hemisphere injury had greater delays than those who had right-hemisphere injuries [45,49]. However, in both samples, the differences were no longer apparent at older ages. In longitudinal studies, there were children in both the left- and right-hemisphere groups who showed normal rates of development and children who were delayed [48,50]. Observation studies of children who had prelinguistic injuries have found no differences in the length and quality of their narrative discourse at school age. The children who had brain injuries made more syntactic errors than the controls in their narratives and their frequency of errors was comparable in the left and right-hemisphere groups [51]. Children who had left-hemisphere injuries had lower scores than children who had other injuries (right-hemisphere lesions and hydrocephalus) on a standardized test of formulating sentences but not on other tests of language functioning, such as following oral directions and recalling sentences [52]. Children from both groups had problems in comparison to their uninjured peers on timed experimental tests of information processing [52]. Both groups were approximately 2 years delayed in comparison to children developing typically on an experimental task that required knowledge of syntax to comprehend sentences [53].

By school age, the mean intelligence quotient for children who have prelingual focal neural injury is generally in the normal range but below the population mean [45,52,54]. The usual pattern of IQ results in adults who have focal brain injury is that left-hemisphere injury lowers the verbal IQ and right-hemisphere injury lowers performance IQ. This pattern is not found in most studies of children who have prelinguistic injuries [54,55].

Taken together, the evidence strongly suggests that left-hemisphere specialization arises in the course of development. The findings argue against a strictly genetic mechanism in favor of activity-dependent cortical specialization. If this is the case, then children who have brain injury should have better outcomes than adults who have comparable injuries. Experimentally, direct comparisons of children and adults who have comparable injuries are inappropriate because children would not be expected to perform at the same level as adults. In addition, the expectations for children vary as a function of age. To get around these methodologic issues, Bates and colleagues [56] compared individual children and adults who had brain injury to appropriate age-matched controls, assigning their performance a z-score based on the mean and standard deviation of the reference sample. The researchers confirmed that children who had early left-hemisphere brain injury had lower z-scores than did adults who had acquired brain injuries, indicating that their performance was closer to the mean for age.

Another implication of developmental specialization is that younger children will have better outcomes after focal injury than older children will. This position, popularized by Lenneberg [57], postulated that the period of plasticity lasted until adolescence. The data confirm the overall premise, but the age at which plasticity declines is not at all clear. For example, in an early study, Woods and Carey [58] found that a younger group who sustained brain injuries at less than 1 year of age had better language outcomes despite mild cognitive deficits than an older group who sustained injuries over 1 year of age. Another early study found age of injury the most important variable in terms of language output, but put the cut-point at age 5 [59]. It is important to realize that not all studies replicate these age effects. For example, Aram and colleagues [60] found that in children who had left-hemisphere injuries in the aftermath of cardiac catheterization or surgery, those who acquired left lesions before 1 year of age did not perform better than those who sustained the injury after 1 year of age on a test of language comprehension. In a more recent study comparing children who had stroke to a comparison group who had orthopedic injuries, the children who had focal injury had persistent difficulties with narrative discourse, and the younger age of injury was associated with greater problems than older age [61].

The good performance of young children who have left-hemisphere focal injuries suggests that their neural organization is different from children developing typically. Functional imaging now offers a noninvasive method to investigate the brain organization in such children. Functional magnetic resonance imaging (fMRI) is the preferred method for functional imaging in children because the technique does not require ionizing radiation [62,63].

Functional MRI capitalizes on two basic phenomena: that increases of neural activity lead to increases of the blood supply, and that oxygenated and unoxygenated hemoglobin have different magnetic properties. Subjects in fMRI studies actively perform tasks, such as comprehending sentences, generating related action words when shown pictures of objects, or reading. The blood oxygenation level–dependent MRI signals during the task are compared with the signals at levels at rest or during other tasks. The technique detects subtle shifts in the hemodynamic patterns across conditions from which the active neural substrate for the function can be inferred.

Typically developing children show increasing left-hemisphere activation for language tasks between ages 7 and 18 [64]. Focal left-hemisphere injury could lead to either constriction of activity within the usual language substrate, expansion of activity to other left-hemisphere regions, or shifts to the right-hemisphere activation during language tasks. Studies find that children who have left-hemisphere brain injury show activation of homologous regions of the right hemisphere during language tasks. One study compared adults, 9- to 12-year-old children developing typically and 9- to 12-year-old children who have neurologic injuries [65,66]. The task required them to understand syntactically complex sentences. A yes–no question after the sentence documented that the subjects were listening and processing the information. Adults were far more accurate at answering the question than were the children, who in turn were more accurate than the children who had brain injury. The typically developing children showed greater left- than right-hemisphere activation during the task, whereas the children who had neurologic injury showed far greater right- than left-hemisphere activation. Another study compared children who had epilepsy from left- and right-hemisphere injuries on a task that required them to silently generate verbs when presented with auditory presentation of nouns [67]. Right-hemisphere lateralization characterized the subjects who had left-hemisphere injury, whereas left-hemisphere activation characterized the children who had right-hemisphere injury. Curiously, right-hemisphere lateralization has been found even in children whose left-hemisphere injuries did not affect classic language areas [67].

Implications

These findings confirm that the cortical brain organization for language is not fixed at birth. It seems to emerge as a function of language learning. It remains unclear why, in the end, most people have left-hemisphere specialization for language. A subtle predisposition for left-hemisphere organization may explain why children who have left-hemisphere injuries are delayed in comparison to children who have right-hemisphere injuries in some studies [49,68]. However, if the left hemisphere is injured, homologous regions of the right hemisphere are capable of serving language functioning. Even if the usual left-hemisphere language areas of the brain are not directly injured, it may be that compromises to the neural flow of information to those regions result in right-hemisphere lateralization. The resulting development, as evidenced by the linguistic performance of children who have prelinguistic injuries, ranges from near normal to moderately impaired.

Several observations suggest that the plasticity of language in the brain may persist beyond the first 3 years of life. At the behavioral level, one study found that a previously nonverbal boy who had Sturge-Webber syndrome began to speak at age 9 after hemispherectomy and withdrawal of anticonvulsant medications. At the neural level, fMRI studies in a boy who had epilepsy from Rasmussen's syndrome documented left-hemisphere lateralization at age 6 and right-hemisphere lateralization at age 9 after left hemispherotomy [69]. Moreover, recovery in adults after left-hemisphere stroke has been shown to correlate with a rightward shift in lateralization during language tasks of fMRI [70]. In the adult study, improvements in performance and rightward shifting of activations occurred within days of the stroke. These findings call into question whether right-hemisphere pathways for language exist in the normal state but are suppressed or overridden in fMRI studies because of greater activity or efficiency of the left hemisphere. Another important area of future research is determining the factors that promote rapid recovery and neural reorganization after early or late brain injuries.

Traumatic brain injury

Findings

Traumatic brain injury results in a combination of diffuse and focal injuries. Diffuse injury results from axonal damage, hypoperfusion, excitotoxic neurotransmitters, and chronic neurotransmitter dysfunction [71]. Focal injury results from the brain striking the skull, the so-called "coup injury," and then ricocheting backward, the so-called "counter-coup damage." There are no studies that directly compare the outcome of children who have focal brain injuries to those who have diffuse injures. Moreover, outcomes of traumatic brain injury vary substantially based on the cause, type, and severity of injuries in addition to the age of injury and years since injury.

Many studies of children who have traumatic injury report speech, language, and discourse sequelae [72–75]. Deficits in the short term after injury may be dramatic, and are followed by variable recovery with persistent long-term problems [76]. Severe injuries are not surprisingly associated with greater long-term difficulties than mild to moderate injuries. However, unlike the patterns after focal injury, younger age at the time of injury is associated with greater deficits than older age [77]. For example, significant deficits in measures of expressive and receptive language were found in young children 2 years after early traumatic brain injury, whereas deficits in lexical functioning were found in only 20% of older children. In the older children, subtle problems, such as word fluency and rapid naming, often persisted [76]. In a longitudinal follow-up study of 122 children who had brain injury and controls, younger age of injury was associated with less favorable outcomes in terms of word fluency than older age [78]. Older children who have severe traumatic brain injury often have striking problems at the level of discourse that compromises their abilities to communicate effectively despite normal syntactic complexity [76]. This pattern is different from that of children who have early focal injury who communicate effectively despite syntactic immaturities. Left-hemisphere focal injury in the context of traumatic brain injury was associated with slowed picture naming, reduced word retrieval, and disruptions of narrative discourse [76].

Implications

Several theorists predict that brain injuries in early life will have greater impact on development than similar injuries in later childhood, particularly for emerging skills [76]. Children who have focal injuries are capable of organizing or reorganizing neural substrate to serve language functions. This contrast implies that there are different pathophysiologic processes in the different conditions. Levin [77] postulates that traumatic brain injury is more likely to disrupt the connections among brain regions accounting for the difficulties in reorganizing neural substrate. The potential for nontraditional areas of brain to serve language may be severely limited if those brain regions cannot communicate effectively with other areas providing input and outflow.

Epilepsy syndromes

Findings

Landau-Kleffner syndrome is a rare clinical condition characterized by the loss of the ability to understand and use spoken language. Behavioral problems, including hyperactivity and irritability, are also common. The condition is associated with epileptiform activity in one or both temporal lobes on electroencephalogram, often occurring at night. Seizures occur in approximately 80% of affected children. However, there are usually no abnormal findings on imaging studies. The condition typically presents between 3 and 7 years of age in children who had been developing normally until that time. The abrupt onset in many cases implicates immune mechanisms [79].

The language problems often continue into adulthood, though some recovery may occur. As in the case of traumatic brain injury, the younger the child is at time of presentation the poorer the prognosis for recovery. No other associations between the extent of language impairment or the presence or absence of seizures and the amount of language recovery have been documented. Some of the children resort to gesturing or succeed at learning sign language, suggesting that the condition affects the phonologic system to a greater extent than other aspects of language and communication. Treatments include anticonvulsant medications, steroids, and individualized education. Some children who have continuous focal epileptiform activity on electroencephalogram have undergone surgical treatment of Landau-Kleffner syndrome. Approximately half of the children show substantial benefits either in terms of language and behavior [80].

Implications

Children who have Landau-Kleffner syndrome are far more impaired than children who have focal brain injury and many children who have traumatic brain injury. If the epileptiform activity directly impaired neural function, it would not explain why after the epileptiform activity resolves, language deficits persist. Another hypothesis is that the epileptiform discharges impair other neural processes, such as synaptic pruning [81]. The epileptiform activity may strengthen syntactic connections that otherwise would have been pruned [82]. A functional imaging study has documented abnormal posterior superior temporal gyral activity in patients who have Landau-Kleffner with persistent symptoms and normal activity in patients who had excellent recovery [83]. Children who have severe epilepsy of other types have better language outcomes than children who have Landau-Kleffner syndrome. In these cases, left-hemisphere seizure foci are associated with reorganization of language functions to the right hemisphere [66,84].

Implications for normal development

This review has used a developmental cognitive neuroscience approach, a review of developmental and linguistic outcomes of various clinical conditions, to investigate requirements for speech and language learning. Studies have demonstrated that access to a rich, varied, and complex verbal environment is vitally important for normal language development (see Table 1). Intermittent minimal to mild conductive hearing loss from otitis media with effusion does not cause serious delays or disorders of speech or language. However, permanent mild to moderate sensorineural hearing loss often leads to phonologic disorders that may be associated with either normal or impaired language functioning and subsequently with normal or abnormal academic skills. Severe and profound hearing loss is associated with poor speech and language skills, though early treatment is associated with improved outcomes. An impoverished verbal environment, which may be associated with poor maternal education or other indicators of low socioeconomic status, is also associated with impairments in vocabulary and syntactic development.

Studies have also shown that though a human brain is necessary for language development (see Table 1), distinct areas of the brain do not appear to be rigidly specialized at the time of birth. There is increasing evidence from animal studies and other clinical conditions that cortical tissue is pluripotential, capable of assuming many different functions under varying circumstances. Children who have early prelinguistic brain injury have good outcomes for conversational speech and language, far better than adults who have comparable injuries. Functional MRI studies find right- rather than left-hemisphere lateralization for language processing after early focal left-hemisphere injury, demonstrating that the behavioral plasticity seems to arise from organization of homologous uninjured brain regions for language functioning. This reorganization occurs in some cases of focal epilepsy. However, severe diffuse brain injury and diffuse severe epileptic syndromes, such as Landau-Kleffner, interferes with plasticity, possibly because of disruption across the connections among brain regions and/or other neural processes such as synaptic pruning.

This plasticity for language functioning in the face of focal injuries may result from the mechanism that allow typically developing children to learn their native language, be it English, Portuguese, or Tagalog. Studies of typically developing infants show that exposure to speech organizes speech perception mechanisms, accounting for a 9-month old infant's declining abilities to differentiate among speech sounds not present in their native language [20]. The human infant as young as 8 months old is sensitive to the statistical regularities that distinguish the recurring sound sequences within words from the more accidental sound sequences between words, even in the absence of intonation and pauses that offer additional information [85]. This ability, which appears to be related to general perceptual abilities, not specific language learning mechanisms, can account for how infants and young children learn to parse the sound stream into the words, phrases, and sentences that they must come to understand and generate [86]. Experience-dependent learning is likely not only organizing abilities at the behavioral level, but also organizing the underlying neural substrates that will serve language functioning. Organizing the neural substrate may be easier when the child is young and has limited perceptual abilities and verbal memory than when the child is older and has committed neural substrate [87]. The importance of experience-dependent learning is most likely the explanation for the powerful effects of access to the verbal environment on the rate of language learning. Limited access on the basis of permanent hearing loss or on the basis of impoverished input can leave an enduring impact on later skills and functioning.

More research is needed to understand the role of environment and neural factors in language learning. Clearly, multiple factors are associated with speech and language outcomes. We have touched on only a few in this review. It is important to learn more about how the role of environment in language learning interacts with neural factors. For example, is the quality of the environment a relevant factor in the degree of plasticity after early focal injuries? Can late enrichment compensate for early deprivation in terms of both behavioral and neural organization? What factors unleash plasticity in older children and adults who have brain injuries?

While we proceed to study further the forces that impact speech and language development, we should also adopt clinical and public policies that maximize children's exposures to rich, interactive verbal environments and that promote healthy neural organization. Improved access to the verbal environment can now be accomplished in cases of hearing loss. In the era of universal newborn hearing screening, it should be routine to get a child with hearing loss amplification by at least 6 months of age if not considerably sooner. An early and aggressive approach to amplification will most likely result in improved outcomes. For children who have severe to profound hearing loss that does not respond favorably to amplification, it is again realistic to make a decision about cochlear implantation by the time the child is 1 year of age, given that research has again demonstrated that early treatment dramatically improves outcomes.

Multiple strategies can be used to improve access to verbal language for children in language-impoverished circumstances. Improving awareness of the importance of verbal input for speech and language outcomes can be accomplished using clinical medicine approaches, such as parent education during child pediatric visits, and by public health approaches, such as public service announcements. Inexpensive parent training should also be readily available. Publicly financed early care and education with well-trained day care providers should also be available, particularly for children living in poverty or under adverse conditions.

We know little about the plasticity of the system as children grow older. Observations of changes in neural organization in school-aged children and adults who have strokes provide optimism that plasticity persists. However, many other observations, such as second-language learning, suggest that our human endowment to learn language deteriorates as we get older. Our clinical and public health strategies for improving access to a rich verbal environment to stimulate neural organization should focus on infants and toddlers but should not ignore interventions with older children who have clinical conditions or early delays and disorders. We must rigorously evaluate the results of all such interventions to refine our understanding of the clinical conditions and at the same time improve children's developmental outcomes.

References

[1] American Speech and Hearing Association. Degree of hearing loss. Available at: http://www.asha.org/public/hearing/disorders/types.htm. Accessed April 1, 2007.

[2] Wake M, Hughes EK, Poulakis Z, et al. Outcomes of children with mild-profound congenital hearing loss at 7 to 8 years: a population study. Ear Hear 2004;25(1):1–8.

[3] Goldin-Meadow S, Feldman H. The development of language-like communication without a language model. Science 1977;197(4301):401–3.

[4] Sandler W, Meir I, Padden C, et al. From the cover: the emergence of grammar: systematic structure in a new language. Proc Natl Acad Sci U S A 2005;102(7):2661–5.

[5] Newport EL. Maturational constraints on language learning. Cognitive Science: A Multidisciplinary Journal 1990;14(1):11–28.

[6] Connor CM, Zwolan TA. Examining multiple sources of influence on the reading comprehension skills of children who use cochlear implants. J Speech Lang Hear Res 2004;47(3): 509–26.

[7] Spencer LJ, Barker BA, Tomblin JB. Exploring the language and literacy outcomes of pediatric cochlear implant users. Ear Hear 2003;24(3):236–47.

[8] Tomblin JB, Spencer LJ, Gantz BJ. Language and reading acquisition in children with and without cochlear implants. Adv Otorhinolaryngol 2000;57:300–4.

[9] Preisler G, Tvingstedt AL, Ahlstrom M. A psychosocial follow-up study of deaf preschool children using cochlear implants. Child Care Health Dev 2002;28(5):403–18.

[10] Chin SB, Tsai PL, Gao S. Connected speech intelligibility of children with cochlear implants and children with normal hearing. Am J Speech Lang Pathol 2003;12(4):440–51.

[11] Eisenberg LS, Kirk KI, Martinez AS, et al. Communication abilities of children with aided residual hearing: comparison with cochlear implant users. Arch Otolaryngol Head Neck Surg 2004;130(5):563–9.

[12] Harrison RV, Gordon KA, Mount RJ. Is there a critical period for cochlear implantation in congenitally deaf children? Analyses of hearing and speech perception performance after implantation. Dev Psychobiol 2005;46(3):252–61.

[13] Rubinstein JT. Paediatric cochlear implantation: prosthetic hearing and language development. Lancet 2002;360(9331):483–5.

[14] Tomblin JB, Barker BA, Spencer LJ, et al. The effect of age at cochlear implant initial stimulation on expressive language growth in infants and toddlers. J Speech Lang Hear Res 2005; 48(4):853–67.

[15] Kovas Y, Hayiou-Thomas ME, Oliver B, et al. Genetic influences in different aspects of language development: the etiology of language skills in 4.5-year-old twins. Child Dev 2005; 76(3):632–51.

[16] Viding E, Spinath FM, Price TS, et al. Genetic and environmental influence on language impairment in 4-year-old same-sex and opposite-sex twins. J Child Psychol Psychiatry 2004; 45(2):315–25.

[17] Shriberg LD, Lewis BA, Tomblin JB, et al. Toward diagnostic and phenotype markers for genetically transmitted speech delay. J Speech Lang Hear Res 2005; 48(4):834–52.

[18] Wake M, Poulakis Z. Slight and mild hearing loss in primary school children. J Paediatr Child Health 2004;40(1–2):11–3.

[19] Briscoe J, Bishop DV, Norbury CF. Phonological processing, language, and literacy: a comparison of children with mild-to-moderate sensorineural hearing loss and those with specific language impairment. J Child Psychol Psychiatry 2001;42(3):329–40.

[20] Kuhl PK. Early language acquisition: cracking the speech code. Nat Rev Neurosci 2004; 5(11):831–43.

[21] Puig T, Municio A, Meda C. Universal neonatal hearing screening versus selective screening as part of the management of childhood deafness. Cochrane Database Syst Rev 2005;2: CD003731.

[22] Yoshinaga-Itano C. Benefits of early intervention for children with hearing loss. Otolaryngol Clin North Am 1999;32(6):1089–102.

[23] Kennedy CR, McCann DC, Campbell MJ, et al. Language ability after early detection of permanent childhood hearing impairment. N Engl J Med 2006;354(20):2131–41.

[24] Sabo DL, Paradise JL, Kurs-Lasky M, et al. Hearing levels in infants and young children in relation to testing technique, age group, and the presence or absence of middle-ear effusion. Ear Hear 2003;24(1):38–47.

[25] Roberts J, Hunter L, Gravel J, et al. Otitis media, hearing loss, and language learning: controversies and current research. J Dev Behav Pediatr 2004;25(2):110–22.

[26] Paradise JL, Rockette HE, Colborn DK, et al. Otitis media in 2253 Pittsburgh-area infants: prevalence and risk factors during the first two years of life. Pediatrics 1997;99(3):318–33.

[27] Paradise JL, Campbell TF, Dollaghan CA, et al. Developmental outcomes after early or delayed insertion of tympanostomy tubes. N Engl J Med 2005;353(6):576–86.

[28] Paradise JL, Feldman HM, Campbell TF, et al. Effect of early or delayed insertion of tympanostomy tubes for persistent otitis media on developmental outcomes at the age of three years. N Engl J Med 2001;344(16):1179–87.

[29] Paradise JL, Feldman HM, Campbell TF, et al. Early versus delayed insertion of tympanostomy tubes for persistent otitis media: developmental outcomes at the age of three years in relation to prerandomization illness patterns and hearing levels. Pediatr Infect Dis J 2003; 22(4):309–14.

[30] Seidenberg MS, MacDonald MC. A probabilistic constraints approach to language acquisition and processing. Cognitive Science 1999;23:569–88.

[31] Dollaghan CA, Campbell TF, Paradise JL, et al. Maternal education and measures of early speech and language. J Speech Lang Hear Res 1999;42(6):1432–43.

[32] Paradise JL, Dollaghan CA, Campbell TF, et al. Language, speech sound production, and cognition in three-year-old children in relation to otitis media in their first three years of life. Pediatrics 2000;105(5):1119–30.

[33] Vasilyeva M, Huttenlocher J, Waterfall H. Effects of language intervention on syntactic skill levels in preschoolers. Dev Psychol 2006;42(1):164–74.

[34] Huttenlocher J, Vasilyeva M, Cymerman E, et al. Language input and child syntax. Cognit Psychol 2002;45(3):337–74.

[35] Huttenlocher J. Language input and language growth. Prev Med 1998;27(2):195–9.

[36] Huttenlocher J, Haight W, Bryk A, et al. Early vocabulary growth: relation to language input and gender. Dev Psychol 1991;27(2):236–48.

[37] Hart B, Risley TR. Meaningful differences in the everyday experiences of young American children. Baltimore (MD): Brookes Publishing Co., Inc.; 1995.

[38] Needlman R, Toker KH, Dreyer BP, et al. Effectiveness of a primary care intervention to support reading aloud: a multicenter evaluation. Ambul Pediatr 2005;5(4):209–15.

[39] Weitzman CC, Roy L, Walls T, et al. More evidence for reach out and read: a home-based study. Pediatrics 2004;113(5):1248–53.

[40] Sharif I, Rieber S, Ozuah PO. Exposure to reach out and read and vocabulary outcomes in inner city preschoolers. J Natl Med Assoc 2002;94(3):171–7.

[41] Keller TA, Carpenter PA, Just MA. The neural bases of sentence comprehension: a fMRI examination of syntactic and lexical processing. Cereb Cortex 2001;11(3): 223–37.

[42] Dall'Oglio AM, Bates E, Volterra V, et al. Early cognition, communication and language in children with focal brain injury. Dev Med Child Neurol 1994;36(12):1076–98.

[43] Marchman VA, Miller R, Bates E. Babble and first words in children with focal brain injury. Appl Psycholinguist 1991;12:1–22.

[44] Bates E, Roe K. Language development in children with unilateral brain injury. In: Nelson CA, Luciana M, editors. Handbook of developmental cognitive neuroscience. Cambridge (MA): MIT Press; 2001. p. 281–307.

[45] Bates E, Thal D, Trauner D, et al. From first words to grammar in children with focal brain injury. Dev Neuropsychol 1997;13:447–76.

[46] Thal D, Marchman V, Stiles J, et al. Early lexical development in children with focal brain injury. Brain Lang 1991;40(4):491–527.

[47] Feldman HM, Holland AL, Kemp SS, et al. Language development after unilateral brain injury. Brain Lang 1992;42(1):89–102.

[48] Feldman HM. Language development after early unilateral brain injury: a replication study. In: Tager-Flusberg H, editor. Constraints on language acquisition: Studies of atypical children. Hillsdale (NJ): Erlbaum; 1994. p. 75–91.

[49] Vicari S, Albertoni A, Chilosi AM, et al. Plasticity and reorganization during language development in children with early brain injury. Cortex 2000;36(1):31–46.

[50] Feldman H, Evans J, Brown R, et al. Early language and communicative abilities of children with periventricular leukomalacia with and without developmental delays. Am J Ment Retard 1992;97:222–34.

[51] Reilly JS, Bates EA, Marchman VA. Narrative discourse in children with early focal brain injury. Brain Lang 1998;61(3):335–75.

[52] MacWhinney B, Feldman H, Sacco K, et al. Online measures of basic language skills in children with early focal brain lesions. Brain Lang 2000;71(3):400–31.

[53] Feldman HM, MacWhinney B, Sacco K. Sentence processing in children with early unilateral brain injury. Brain Lang 2002;83(2):335–52.

[54] Vargha-Khadem F, Isaacs E, Watkins K, et al. Ontogentic specialization of hemispheric function. In: Polkey CE, Duchowney M, editors. Intractable focal epilepsy: medical and surgical treatment. London: Harcourt Publishers; 2000. p. 405–18.

[55] Bates E, Vicari S, Trauner D. Neural mediation of language development: perspectives from lesion studies of infants and children. In: Tager-Flusberg H, editor. Neurodevelopmental disorders. Cambridge (MA): MIT Press; 1999. p. 533–81.

[56] Bates E, Reilly J, Wulfeck B, et al. Differential effects of unilateral lesions on language production in children and adults. Brain Lang 2001;79(2):223–65.

[57] Lenneberg EH. Biological foundations of language. New York: Wiley; 1967.

[58] Woods BT, Carey S. Language deficits after apparent clinical recovery from childhood aphasia. Ann Neurol 1979;6(5):405–9.

[59] Vargha-Khadem F, O'Gorman AM, Watters GV. Aphasia and handedness in relation to hemispheric side, age at injury and severity of cerebral lesion during childhood. Brain 1985;108(Pt 3):677–96.

[60] Aram DM, Ekelman BL. Unilateral brain lesions in childhood: performance on the Revised Token Test. Brain & Language 1987;32(1):137–58.

[61] Chapman SB, Max JE, Gamino JF, et al. Discourse plasticity in children after stroke: age at injury and lesion effects. Pediatr Neurol 2003;29(1):34–41.

[62] Logan WJ. Functional magnetic resonance imaging in children. Semin Pediatr Neurol 1999; 6(2):78–86.

[63] Hertz-Pannier L, Gaillard WD, Mott SH, et al. Noninvasive assessment of language dominance in children and adolescents with functional MRI: a preliminary study. Neurology 1997;48(4):1003–12.

[64] Holland SK, Plante E, Weber Byars A, et al. Normal fMRI brain activation patterns in children performing a verb generation task. Neuroimage 2001;14(4):837–43.

[65] Booth JR, Macwhinney B, Thulborn KR, et al. Functional organization of activation patterns in children: whole brain fMRI imaging during three different cognitive tasks. Prog Neuropsychopharmacol Biol Psychiatry 1999;23(4):669–82.

[66] Booth JR, MacWhinney B, Thulborn KR, et al. Developmental and lesion effects in brain activation during sentence comprehension and mental rotation. Dev Neuropsychol 2000; 18(2):139–69.

[67] Liegeois F, Connelly A, Cross JH, et al. Language reorganization in children with early-onset lesions of the left hemisphere: an fMRI study. Brain 2004;127(Pt 6):1229–36.

[68] Bates E, Elman J. The ontogeny and phylogeny of language: a neural network perspective. In: Parker ST, Langer J, McKinney M, editors. Biology, brains, and behavior: the evolution of human development. Santa Fe (NM): School of American Research Press; 2000. p. 89–130.

[69] Hertz-Pannier L, Chiron C, Jambaque I, et al. Late plasticity for language in a child's non-dominant hemisphere: a pre- and post-surgery fMRI study. Brain 2002;125(Pt 2): 361–72.

[70] Thulborn KR, Carpenter PA, Just MA. Plasticity of language-related brain function during recovery from stroke. Stroke 1999;30(4):749–54.

[71] Adelson PD, Kochanek PM. Head injury in children. J Child Neurol 1998;13(1):2–15.

[72] Moran C, Gillon G. Language and memory profiles of adolescents with traumatic brain injury. Brain Inj 2004;18(3):273–88.

[73] Catroppa C, Anderson V. Recovery and predictors of language skills two years following pediatric traumatic brain injury. Brain Lang 2004;88(1):68–78.

[74] Chapman SB, McKinnon L, Levin HS, et al. Longitudinal outcome of verbal discourse in children with traumatic brain injury: three-year follow-up. J Head Trauma Rehabil 2001; 16(5):441–55.

[75] Campbell TF, Dollaghan CA. Speaking rate, articulatory speed, and linguistic processing in children and adolescents with severe traumatic brain injury. J Speech Hear Res 1995;38(4): 864–75.

[76] Ewing-Cobbs L, Barnes M. Linguistic outcomes following traumatic brain injury in children. Semin Pediatr Neurol 2002;9(3):209–17.

[77] Levin HS. Neuroplasticity following non-penetrating traumatic brain injury. Brain Inj 2003; 17(8):665–74.

[78] Levin HS, Song J, Ewing-Cobbs L, et al. Word fluency in relation to severity of closed head injury, associated frontal brain lesions, and age at injury in children. Neuropsychologia 2001; 39(2):122–31.

[79] Boscolo S, Baldas V, Gobbi G, et al. Anti-brain but not celiac disease antibodies in Landau-Kleffner syndrome and related epilepsies. J Neuroimmunol 2005;160(1–2):228–32.

[80] Mikati MA, Shamseddine AN. Management of Landau-Kleffner syndrome. Paediatr Drugs 2005;7(6):377–89.

[81] Honbolygo F, Csepe V, Fekeshazy A, et al. Converging evidences on language impairment in Landau-Kleffner syndrome revealed by behavioral and brain activity measures: a case study. Clin Neurophysiol 2006;117(2):295–305.

[82] Smith MC, Hoeppner TJ. Epileptic encephalopathy of late childhood: Landau-Kleffner syndrome and the syndrome of continuous spikes and waves during slow-wave sleep. J Clin Neurophysiol 2003;20(6):462–72.

[83] Majerus S, Laureys S, Collette F, et al. Phonological short-term memory networks following recovery from Landau and Kleffner syndrome. Hum Brain Mapp 2003;19(3):133–44.

[84] Yuan W, Szaflarski JP, Schmithorst VJ, et al. fMRI shows atypical language lateralization in pediatric epilepsy patients. Epilepsia 2006;47(3):593–600.

[85] Saffran JR, Aslin RN, Newport EL. Statistical learning by 8-month-old infants. Science 1996;274(5294):1926–8.

[86] Saffran JR, Johnson EK, Aslin RN, et al. Statistical learning of tone sequences by human infants and adults. Cognition 1999;70(1):27–52.

[87] Elman JL. Learning and development in neural networks: the importance of starting small. Cognition 1993;48(1):71–99.

PEDIATRIC CLINICS

OF NORTH AMERICA

ELSEVIER
SAUNDERS

Pediatr Clin N Am 54 (2007) 609–623

Management of Dyslexia, Its Rationale, and Underlying Neurobiology

Sally E. Shaywitz, MD[a,b,]*, Jeffrey R. Gruen, MD[c],
Bennett A. Shaywitz, MD[a,b]

[a]Department of Pediatrics, Division of Child Neurology, Yale University School of Medicine,
PO Box 333, New Haven, CT 06510–8064, USA
[b]Yale Center for the Study of Learning, Reading, and Attention, Yale University School
of Medicine, PO Box 333, New Haven, CT 06510–8064, USA
[c]Department of Pediatrics, Division of Neonatology, Yale University School of Medicine,
PO Box 333, New Haven, CT 06510–8064, USA

Developmental dyslexia is characterized by an unexpected difficulty in reading in children and adults who otherwise possess the intelligence and motivation considered necessary for accurate and fluent reading [1–5]. Dyslexia (or specific reading disability) is the most common and most carefully studied of the learning disabilities, affecting 80% of all individuals identified as learning disabled. Although in the past the diagnosis and implications of dyslexia were often uncertain, recent advances in the knowledge of the epidemiology, the neurobiology, the genetics, and the cognitive influences on the disorder now allow the disorder to be approached within the framework of a traditional medical model. This article reviews these advances and their implications for the approach to patients presenting with a possible reading disability.

Epidemiology

Epidemiologic data indicate that, like hypertension and obesity, dyslexia occurs in gradations and fits a dimensional model. Within the population,

---

The work described was supported by grants from the National Institute of Child Health and Human Development (PO1 HD 21888 and P50 HD25802) to Bennett and Sally Shaywitz, and from the National Institute of Neurological Disease and Stroke (R01 NS 43530) to Jeffrey Gruen. Portions of this article have appeared whole or in part elsewhere [1–5].

* Corresponding author. Department of Pediatrics, Division of Child Neurology, Yale University School of Medicine, PO Box 333, New Haven, CT 06510–8064.

E-mail address: sally.shaywitz@yale.edu (S.E. Shaywitz).

reading ability and reading disability occur along a continuum, with reading disability representing the lower tail of a normal distribution of reading ability [6,7]. Dyslexia is perhaps the most common neurobehavioral disorder affecting children, with prevalence rates ranging from 5% to 17.5% [2,8]. Although some may question whether so many children are struggling to read, data from the 2005 National Assessment of Educational Progress [9] indicate that only 31% of fourth graders are performing at or above proficient levels. Dyslexia does not resolve over time. Longitudinal studies, both prospective [10,11] and retrospective [12–14], indicate that dyslexia is a persistent, chronic condition; it does not represent a transient developmental lag (Fig. 1). Over time, poor readers and good readers tend to maintain their relative positions along the spectrum of reading ability [10,15]; children who early on function at the tenth percentile for reading and those who function at the 90% percentile and all those in-between tend to maintain their positions.

Etiology

Dyslexia is both familial and heritable [16]. Family history is one of the most important risk factors, with 23% to as much as 65% of children who have a parent with dyslexia reported to have the disorder [14]. A rate among siblings of affected persons of approximately 40% and among parents ranging from 27% to 49% [16] provides opportunities for early identification of affected siblings and often for delayed but helpful identification of affected adults, such as a parent of the child known to be dyslexic. Despite the strong familial nature, within a single family both recessive and dominant transmission is frequently observed. These data are consistent with a complex etiology; studies of heritability show that between 44% and 75% of the variance is explained by genetic factors and the remaining by environmental factors [17].

These genetic factors are sequence variations of several genes (ie, polygenic) that act in concert to produce the dyslexia phenotype, and because of the polygenic nature, create confusing transmission patterns that do not follow traditional mendelian rules governing recessive, dominant, or sex-linked single-gene disorders. Regardless of these complexities, genetic linkage studies, enabled in large part by the achievements of the Human Genome Project, have identified broad locations on human chromosomes, called loci, where dyslexia genes are encoded. To date, a total of nine loci have been identified, named "DYX1" through "DYX9" for the order in which they were recognized, and have been cataloged as official "DYX" loci in the Online Mammalian Inheritance in Man database.

Of the nine described dyslexia loci, the most widely reproduced has been DYX2 located on the "p" or short arm of chromosome 6 in band "22" (6p22), spanning nearly 20 million bases. Recently, the authors reported association of the DCDC2 gene encoded on 6p22 with several reading-related

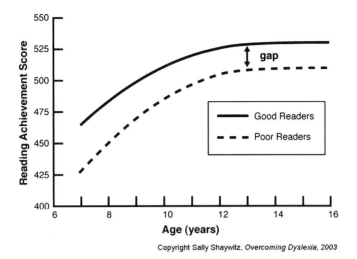

Copyright Sally Shaywitz, *Overcoming Dyslexia, 2003*

Fig. 1. Trajectory of reading skills over time in nonimpaired and dyslexic readers. Ordinate is Rasch scores (W scores) from the Woodcock-Johnson reading test [54] and abscissa is age in years. Both dyslexic and nonimpaired readers improve their reading scores as they get older, but the gap between the dyslexic and nonimpaired readers remains. Dyslexia is a deficit and not a developmental lag. (*From* Shaywitz S. Overcoming dyslexia: a new and complete science-based program for reading problems at any level. New York: Alfred Knopf; 2003. p. 34; with permission.)

phenotypes, suggesting a specific effect on reading performance [18]. Further, in human brain, DCDC2 expression correlated with the location of reading-related brain systems (see later), and it was found that DCDC2 in rats modulated neuronal migration. The association between DCDC2 and dyslexia was subsequently and independently confirmed by Schumacher and colleagues [19] in a two-tiered study of 137 and 239 families with dyslexia from Germany, thereby validating the findings and the universality of the genetic effect across languages and cultures.

Other candidate genes for dyslexia have been described. Encoded just 500,000 bases away from DCDC2, Cope and colleagues [20] described a second candidate gene for DYX2, called KIAA0319, which in 143 families from the United Kingdom also contributed to dyslexia. Two other candidates, EKN1 (DYX1) and ROBO1 (DYX5), were identified by cloning rare translocation breakpoints in single families from Finland, but validation in additional populations would make for more convincing evidence [21,22]. Gene discovery for all the dyslexia loci remains an active area of study.

Cognitive influences

Among investigators in the field, there is now a strong consensus supporting the phonologic theory. This theory recognizes that speech is natural and inherent, whereas reading is acquired and must be taught. To read, the beginning reader must recognize that the letters and letter strings (the orthography) represent the sounds of spoken language. To read, a child has to develop the insight that spoken words can be pulled apart into the elemental particles of speech (phonemes) and that the letters in a written word represent these sounds [3]; such awareness is largely missing in dyslexic children and adults [3,12,23–27]. Results from large and well-studied populations with reading disability confirm that in young school-age children [23,28] and in adolescents [29], a deficit in phonology represents the most robust and specific correlate of reading disability [30,31]. Such findings form the basis for the most successful and evidence-based interventions designed to improve reading [32].

Neurobiologic studies of disabled readers

Neural systems influencing reading were first proposed over a century ago by Dejerine [33] in studies of adults who suffered a stroke with subsequent acquired alexia, the sudden loss of the ability to read. It has only been within the last two decades that neuroscientists have been able to determine the neural systems that influence reading and reading disability. This explosion in understanding the neural bases of reading and dyslexia has been driven by the development of functional neuroimaging, techniques that measure changes in metabolic activity and blood flow in specific brain regions while subjects are engaged in cognitive tasks. These technologies include positron emission tomography and functional MRI; both depend on the principle of autoregulation of cerebral blood flow. Details of functional MRI are reviewed elsewhere [34–36].

A number of research groups have used positron emission tomography or functional MRI to examine the functional organization of the brain for reading in nonimpaired and dyslexic readers, and generally have validated these two left hemisphere posterior systems as critical to reading. For example, in studies of adults [37] and in a study of 144 children, half of whom were struggling readers and half nonimpaired readers, the authors [38] found significant differences in brain activation patterns during phonologic analysis between dyslexic and nonimpaired children. Specifically, nonimpaired children demonstrate significantly greater activation than dyslexic children in predominantly left hemisphere sites (including the inferior frontal, superior temporal, parietotemporal, and middle temporal–middle occipital gyri). These data converge with reports that show a failure of left hemisphere posterior brain systems to function properly during reading and indicate that dysfunction in left hemisphere posterior reading circuits is already present in dyslexic children and cannot be ascribed simply to a lifetime of poor reading [5,39]. Although dyslexic readers exhibit a dysfunction in posterior reading systems, they seem to develop compensatory systems involving areas around the inferior frontal gyrus in both hemispheres and the right hemisphere homolog of the left occipitotemporal word form area [38].

These studies indicate that in addition to the posterior systems, an anterior system is also involved in reading. The anterior network in the inferior frontal gyrus (Broca's area) has long been associated with articulation and also serves an important function in silent reading and naming [35,40]. The two posterior regions seem to parallel the two systems proposed by Logan [41,42] as critical in the development of skilled, automatic reading. One system involves word analysis; operates on individual units of words, such as phonemes; requires attentional resources; and processes information relatively slowly. It is reasonable to propose that this system involves the parietotemporal posterior reading network. Considerable research in the last 5 years has converged to indicate that the second posterior network, localized to a region termed the "visual word-form area" [43], influences skilled, fluent reading. Dehaene and associates [44–46] have suggested a systematic sensitivity to coding within the left occipitotemporal region, with more posterior regions coding for letters and letter fragments and more anterior regions coding for bigrams and words. Furthermore, recent evidence indicates that the disruption in the left occipitotemporal word form area in dyslexic individuals is found not only for reading words, but for naming the pictures of the words, suggesting that the disruption in this region "reflects a more general impairment in retrieving phonology from visual input. In other words, reduced activation in the same occipitotemporal region may underlie the reading and naming deficits observed in developmental dyslexia" (Fig. 2) [47].

Functional MRI has been helpful in clarifying potentially different types of reading disability [3]. The authors used data from the Connecticut Longitudinal Study, a representative sample of now young adults who have been prospectively followed since 1983 when they were age 5 years and who have had their reading performance assessed yearly throughout their primary and secondary schooling. Three groups were identified and imaged: (1) nonimpaired readers who had no evidence of reading problems; (2) accuracy improved readers (AIR) who were inaccurate readers in third grade but by ninth grade had compensated to some degree so they were accurate (but not fluent); and (3) persistently poor readers (PPR) who were inaccurate readers in third grade and remained inaccurate and not fluent in ninth grade.

During real word reading, brain activation patterns in the two groups of disabled readers (AIR and PPR) diverged, with AIR demonstrating the typical disruption of posterior systems, but with PPR activating posterior systems, similar to that observed in nonimpaired readers, despite the significantly better reading performance in nonimpaired readers compared with PPR on every reading task administered. Evidence indicated that rather than decoding words, the PPR group was reading primarily by memory. Because it is a longitudinal study, data from the Connecticut

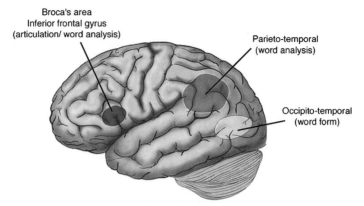

Copyright Sally Shaywitz, *Overcoming Dyslexia, 2003*

Fig. 2. Neural systems for reading. Three neural systems for reading are illustrated in this figure of the surface of the left hemisphere: an anterior system in the region of the inferior frontal gyrus (Broca's area) believed to serve articulation and word analysis; two posterior systems, one in the parieto-temporal region believed to serve word analysis, and a second in the occipito-temporal region (termed the "word-form" area) and believed to serve for the rapid, automatic, fluent identification of words. (*From* Shaywitz S. Overcoming dyslexia: a new and complete science-based program for reading problems at any level. New York: Alfred Knopf; 2003. p. 78; with permission.)

Longitudinal Study as early as kindergarten and first grade were available and indicated that the two groups of disabled readers (PPR and AIR) began school with comparable reading skills but with PPR compared with AIR having poorer cognitive, primarily verbal, ability and attending more disadvantaged schools.

These and other findings suggest that PPR may be doubly disadvantaged in being exposed to a less rich language environment at home and then less effective reading instruction at school. In contrast, the presence of compensatory factors, such as stronger verbal ability and exposure to a richer language environment at home, allowed the AIR to minimize, in part, the consequences of their phonologic deficit so that as adults AIR were indistinguishable from nonimpaired readers on a measure of reading comprehension.

These findings of differences, neurobiologically, cognitively, and educationally, suggest that the two types of reading disability observed in the Connecticut Longitudinal sample may represent different etiologies. The compensated group (AIR), with early higher verbal ability and a disruption in posterior systems during reading real words, may represent a primarily genetic type of reading disability; one can postulate that such children represent the classic dyslexic reader with an unexpected difficulty in reading. Alternatively, the persistent group (PPR), who score lower on verbal measures early on and who attend more disadvantaged schools, may have their reading difficulties influenced more by environmental factors. Other factors also may be operating. Ongoing studies of genetic differences between these groups may help confirm or refute this hypothesis.

Functional imaging has been helpful in examining whether the neural systems for reading are malleable and whether the disruption in these systems in struggling readers can be modified by an effective reading intervention. Compared with struggling readers who received other types of intervention, children who received an experimental intervention not only improved their reading but, compared with preintervention brain imaging, demonstrated increased activation in the neural systems for reading [48]. Other investigators also have found that an effective reading intervention influences neural systems in brain [5]. These data have important implications for public policy regarding teaching children to read: the provision of an evidence-based reading intervention at an early age improves reading fluency and facilitates the development of those neural systems that underlie skilled reading.

Diagnosis

At all ages, dyslexia is a clinical diagnosis. The clinician seeks to determine through history, observation, and psychometric assessment if there are unexpected difficulties in reading (ie, difficulties in reading that are unexpected for the person's age, intelligence, or level of education or professional status), and associated linguistic problems at the level of phonologic processing. There is no one single test score that is pathognomonic of dyslexia. As with any other medical diagnosis, the diagnosis of dyslexia should reflect a thoughtful synthesis of all the available clinical data. Dyslexia is distinguished from other disorders that may prominently feature reading difficulties by the unique, circumscribed nature of the phonologic deficit, one not intruding into other linguistic or cognitive domains.

In the preschool child, a history of language-delay or of not attending to the sounds of words (trouble learning nursery rhymes or playing rhyming games with words, confusing words that sound alike, mispronouncing words), trouble learning to recognize the letters of the alphabet, along with a positive family history represent important risk factors for dyslexia. In the school-aged child, presenting complaints most commonly center about school performance ("she's not doing well in school"), and often parents (and teachers) do not appreciate that the reason for this is a reading difficulty. A typical picture is that of a child who may have had a delay in speaking, does not learn letters by kindergarten, has not begun to learn to read by first grade, and has difficulty consistently sounding out words. The child progressively falls behind, with teachers and parents puzzled as to why such an intelligent child may have difficulty learning to read. The reading difficulty is unexpected with respect to the child's ability, age, or grade. Even after acquiring decoding skills, the child generally remains a slow reader. Bright dyslexic children may laboriously learn how to read words accurately but do not become fluent readers (ie, they do not recognize words rapidly and automatically). Dysgraphia and spelling difficulties are often present, and accompanied by laborious notetaking. Self-esteem is frequently affected, particularly if the disorder has gone undetected for a long period of time (Table 1) [3].

In an accomplished adolescent or young adult, dyslexia is often reflected by slowness in reading or choppy reading aloud that is unexpected in relation to the level of education or professional status (eg, graduation from a competitive college or completion of medical school and a residency). In bright adolescents and young adults, a history of phonologically based reading difficulties, requirements for extra time on tests, and current slow and effortful reading (ie, signs of a lack of automaticity in reading), are the sine qua non of a diagnosis of dyslexia. At all ages, a history of difficulties getting to the basic sounds of spoken language, of laborious and slow reading and writing, of poor spelling, of requiring additional time in reading and in taking tests, provide indisputable evidence of a deficiency in phonologic processing, which in turn serves as the basis for, and the signature of, a reading disability.

Assessment of prereading and reading

Even before the time a child is expected to read, a child's readiness to read may be assessed by measurement of the skills, especially phonologic, related to reading success. Following a predictable developmental pathway,

Table 1
Clues to dyslexia in the school-age child

Problems in speaking
  • Mispronunciation of long or complicated words
  • Speech that is not fluent—pausing or hesitating often
  • Use of imprecise language
Problems in reading
  • Very slow progress in acquiring reading skills
  • The lack of a strategy to read new words
  • Trouble reading unknown (new, unfamiliar) words sounded out
  • The inability to read small function words, such as that, an, in
  • Oral reading that is choppy and labored
  • Disproportionately poor performance on multiple-choice tests
  • The inability to finish tests on time
  • Disastrous spelling
  • Reading that is very slow and tiring
  • Messy handwriting
  • Extreme difficulty learning a foreign language
  • History of reading, spelling, and foreign language problems in family members

From Shaywitz S. Overcoming dyslexia: a new and complete science-based program for reading problems at any level. New York: Alfred Knopf; 2003. p. 223; with permission.

children's phonologic abilities can be evaluated beginning at about age 4 years. Mainly, such tests are centered on a child's ability to focus, initially on syllables, and later on phonemes, the basic particles of spoken language. Initial tests typically ask what word rhymes with another or what spoken word begins (or ends) with the same sound as another. At more advanced levels, tests ask children to pronounce a spoken word after a sound is removed; for example, "can you say steak without the "t" sound (sake)" or "can you count the number of sounds you hear in man (three sounds: 'mmmm'....'aaaa'...'nnn')." In general, as a child develops, he or she gains the ability to notice and to manipulate smaller and smaller parts of spoken words. Tests of phonologic capabilities and reading readiness are becoming increasingly available; one such test is the Comprehensive Test of Phonological Processing in Reading, nationally standardized for age 5 through adult years [49]. In addition to phonology, knowledge of letter names and sounds are the strongest predictors of a child's readiness to read. An appropriate battery of tests for the early recognition of reading problems includes tests of phonology, letter names and sounds, vocabulary, print conventions, and listening comprehension. Tests of reading are also useful because they allow comparison of a child's reading skills with his or her peers at a time when one should be beginning to read [3]. It is important to note that tests of intelligence are relatively poor predictors of later reading difficulties or of response to reading interventions. The importance of such early assessments is that they can identify at-risk children early on so that these boys and girls can be provided with the highly effective, evidence-based reading interventions now available.

Reading is assessed by measuring decoding (accuracy); fluency; and comprehension. In the school-age child, one important element of the evaluation is how accurately the child can decode words (ie, read single words in isolation). This is measured with standardized tests of single real word and pseudoword reading, such as the Woodcock-Johnson III [50] and the Woodcock Reading Mastery Tests [51]. Pseudoword reading, measuring the ability to decode nonsense or made-up words, is a particularly useful test. Because the words are made-up, the child has not seen them before and could not have memorized the words; each nonsense word must be sounded out. Tests of nonsense word reading are referred to as "word attack." Silent reading comprehension may be assessed by either Woodcock test. Reading fluency, the ability to read accurately, rapidly, and with good intonation, is a critical but often overlooked component of reading. The ability to read words fluently is an indication that these words are read automatically, without the need to apply attentional resources. Fluency is generally assessed by asking the child to read aloud using the Gray Oral Reading Test [52]. This test consists of 13 increasingly difficult passages, each followed by five comprehension questions; scores for accuracy, rate, fluency, and comprehension are provided. Such tests of oral reading are particularly helpful in identifying a child who is dyslexic; by its nature oral reading forces a child to pronounce each word. Listening to a struggling reader attempt to pronounce each word leaves no doubt about the child's reading difficulty. In addition to reading passages aloud, single word reading efficiency may be assessed using the Test of Word Reading Efficiency, a test of speeded oral reading of individual words [53]. Children who struggle with reading often have trouble spelling. In reading, the written word is decoded into its constituent sounds; in spelling, sounds in a spoken word are encoded into letters. The Wide Range Achievement Test [54] and the Test of Written Spelling-4 [55] are among the tests that measure spelling.

For informal screening by primary care physicians in an office setting the authors recommend listening to the child read aloud from his or her own grade level reader. Keeping a set of graded readers available in the office serves the purpose and does not require the child to bring in their own school books. Oral reading is a very sensitive measure of not only reading accuracy, but even more importantly, reading fluency.

The most consistent and telling sign of a reading disability in an accomplished young adult is slow and laborious reading and writing. It must be emphasized that the failure either to recognize or to measure the lack of automaticity in reading is perhaps the most common error in the diagnosis of dyslexia in older children and in accomplished young adults. Simple word identification tasks do not detect a dyslexic accomplished enough to be in honors high school classes or to graduate from college and attend law, medical, or any other graduate degree school. Tests relying on the accuracy of word identification alone are inappropriate to use to diagnose dyslexia in accomplished young adults; tests of word identification reveal little to nothing of their struggles to read. It is important to recognize that, because they assess reading accuracy but not automaticity (speed), the kinds of reading tests commonly used for school-age children may provide misleading data on bright adolescents and young adults. The most critical tests are those that are timed; they are the most sensitive to a phonologic deficit in a bright adult. There are very few standardized tests for young adult readers, however, that are administered under timed and untimed conditions; the Nelson-Denny Reading Test represents an exception [56]. Any scores obtained on testing must be considered relative to peers with the same degree of education or professional training.

Developmental course and outcome

Deficits in phonologic coding continue to characterize dyslexic readers even in adolescence; performance on phonologic processing measures contributes most to discriminating dyslexic and average adolescent readers, and also average and superior adolescent readers [29]. Children with dyslexia neither spontaneously remit, nor do they demonstrate, a lag mechanism for "catching up" in the development of reading skills. Many dyslexic readers may become quite proficient in reading a finite domain of words that recur over and over again in their area of special interest, usually words that are important for their careers. For example, an individual who is dyslexic in childhood but who in adult life becomes interested in molecular biology may then learn to decode words that form a minivocabulary important in molecular biology. Such an individual, although able to decode words in this domain, still exhibits evidence of early reading problems when they have to read unfamiliar words, which they then read accurately but not fluently and automatically [12,29,57–59]. Because they are able to read words accurately (albeit very slowly), dyslexic adolescents and young adults may mistakenly be assumed to have "outgrown" their dyslexia. Data from studies of children with dyslexia who have been followed prospectively support the notion that in adolescents, the rate of reading and facility with spelling may be most useful clinically in differentiating average from poor readers in students in secondary school, and college and even graduate school. It is important to remember that these older dyslexic students may be similar to their unimpaired peers on untimed measures of word recognition, yet continue to suffer from the phonologic deficit that makes reading less automatic, more effortful, and slow. For these readers with dyslexia the provision of extra time is an essential accommodation; it allows them the time to decode each word and to apply their unimpaired higher-order cognitive and linguistic skills to the surrounding context to get at the meaning of words that they cannot entirely or rapidly decode. Other accommodations useful to adolescents with reading difficulties include note-takers; taping classroom lectures; using Recordings for the Blind to access texts and other books they have difficulty reading; and the opportunity to take tests in alternate formats, such as short essays [3].

Reading instruction and intervention

The management of dyslexia demands a life span perspective; early on, the focus is on remediation of the reading problem. As a child matures and enters the more time-demanding setting of secondary school, the emphasis shifts to incorporate the important role of providing accommodations. Effective intervention programs provide children with systematic instruction in each of five critical components of reading: (1) phonemic awareness (the ability to focus on and manipulate phonemes, speech sounds, in spoken syllables and words); (2) phonics (understanding how letters are linked to sounds to form letter-sound correspondences and spelling patterns); (3) fluency; (4) vocabulary; and (5) comprehension strategies. The goal is for children to develop the skills that allow them to read and understand the meaning of both familiar and unfamiliar words they may encounter. Large-scale studies to date have focused on younger children; as yet, there are few or no data available on the effect of these training programs on older children. The data on younger children are extremely encouraging, indicating that using evidence-based methods can remediate, and may even prevent, reading difficulties in primary school-aged children [3,60,61].

An essential component of the management of dyslexia in students in secondary school, and especially college and graduate school, incorporates the provision of accommodations. High school and college students with a history of childhood dyslexia often present a paradoxical picture; they are similar to their unimpaired peers on measures of word recognition and comprehension, yet continue to suffer from the phonologic deficit that makes reading less automatic, more effortful, and slow. Neurobiologic data now provide strong evidence for the necessity of extra time for readers with dyslexia. Functional MRI data demonstrate a disruption in the word form area, the region supporting rapid reading. At the same time, readers compensate by developing anterior systems bilaterally and the right homolog of the left word form area. Such compensation allows for accurate reading, but does not support fluent or rapid reading [38]. Consequently, for these readers with dyslexia the provision of extra time is an essential accommodation; it allows them the time to decode each word and to apply their unimpaired higher-order cognitive and linguistic skills to the surrounding context to get at the meaning of words that they cannot entirely or rapidly decode. With such accommodations, many students with dyslexia are now successfully completing studies in a range of disciplines, including medicine.

People with dyslexia and their families frequently consult their physicians about unconventional approaches to the remediation of reading difficulties; in general, there are very few credible data to support the claims made for these treatments (eg, optometric training, medication for vestibular dysfunction, chiropractic manipulation, and dietary supplementation). Finally, pediatricians should be aware that there is no one "magical" program that remediates reading difficulties; a number of programs following the guidelines provided previously have proved to be highly effective in teaching struggling children to read.

Summary

Within the last two decades overwhelming evidence from many laboratories has converged to indicate the cognitive basis for dyslexia: dyslexia represents a disorder within the language system and more specifically within a particular subcomponent of that system, phonologic processing. Recent advances in imaging technology and the development of tasks that sharply isolate the subcomponent processes of reading now allow the localization of phonologic processing in brain, and as a result provide for the first time the potential for elucidating a biologic signature for reading and reading disability. Converging evidence from a number of laboratories using functional brain imaging indicates a disruption of left hemisphere posterior brain systems in child and adult dyslexic readers while performing reading tasks with an additional suggestion for an associated increased reliance on ancillary systems (eg, in the frontal lobes and right hemisphere posterior circuits). The discovery of neural systems serving reading has significant implications. At the most fundamental level, it is now possible to investigate specific hypotheses regarding the neural substrate of dyslexia, and to verify, reject, or modify suggested cognitive models. From a more clinical perspective, the identification of neural systems for reading has implications for the acceptance of dyslexia as a valid disorder, a necessary condition for its identification and treatment. They provide, for the first time, convincing, irrefutable evidence that what has been considered a hidden disability is real. Such findings should make policy makers more willing to allow children and adolescents with dyslexia to receive accommodations on high stakes tests, such accommodations as extra time, which allow dyslexic readers with a disruption in the word form area influencing skilled, fluent reading, to be on a level playing field with their peers who do not have a reading disability.

References

[1] Shaywitz S, Shaywitz B. Dyslexia. In: Swaiman K, Ashwal S, Ferriero D, editors. Pediatric neurology: principles and practice. 4th edition. St. Louis (MO): Mosby Elsevier; 2006. p. 857–70.

[2] Shaywitz S. Current concepts: dyslexia. N Engl J Med 1998;338(5):307–12.

[3] Shaywitz S. Overcoming dyslexia: a new and complete science-based program for reading problems at any level. New York: Alfred A. Knopf; 2003.

[4] Shaywitz S, Shaywitz B. Dyslexia: specific reading disability. Pediatr Rev 2003;24:147–53.

[5] Shaywitz S, Shaywitz B. Dyslexia (specific reading disability). Biol Psychiatry 2005;57: 1301–9.

[6] Gilger JW, Borecki IB, Smith SD, et al. The etiology of extreme scores for complex phenotypes: an illustration using reading performance. In: Chase CH, Rosen GD, Sherman GF, editors. Developmental dyslexia: neural, cognitive, and genetic mechanisms. Baltimore (MD): York Press; 1996. p. 63–85.

[7] Shaywitz SE, Escobar MD, Shaywitz BA, et al. Evidence that dyslexia may represent the lower tail of a normal distribution of reading ability. N Engl J Med 1992;326(3):145–50.

[8] Interagency Committee on Learning Disabilities. Learning disabilities: a report to the U.S. Congress. Washington, DC: U.S. Government Printing Office; 1987.

[9] Perie M, Grigg W, Donahue P. The nation's report card: reading 2005. In: U.S. Department of Education IoES, National Center for Education Statistics, editor. Washington, DC: U.S. Government Printing Office; 2005.

[10] Francis DJ, Shaywitz SE, Stuebing KK, et al. Developmental lag versus deficit models of reading disability: a longitudinal, individual growth curves analysis. J Educ Psychol 1996; 88(1):3–17.

[11] Shaywitz BA, Fletcher JM, Holahan JM, et al. Interrelationships between reading disability and attention-deficit/hyperactivity disorder. Child Neuropsychol 1995;1(3):170–86.

[12] Bruck M. Persistence of dyslexics' phonological awareness deficits. Dev Psychol 1992;28(5): 874–86.

[13] Felton RH, Naylor CE, Wood FB. Neuropsychological profile of adult dyslexics. Brain Lang 1990;39:485–97.

[14] Scarborough HS. Very early language deficits in dyslexic children. Child Dev 1990;61:1728–43.

[15] Shaywitz BA, Holford TR, Holahan JM, et al. A Matthew effect for IQ but not for reading: results from a longitudinal study. Reading Research Quarterly 1995;30(4):894–906.

[16] Pennington BF, Gilger JW. How is dyslexia transmitted? In: Chase CH, Rosen GD, Sherman GF, editors. Developmental dyslexia: neural, cognitive, and genetic mechanisms. Baltimore (MD): York Press; 1996. p. 41–61.

[17] DeFries JC, Olson RK, Pennington BF, et al. Colorado reading project: an update. In: Duane DD, Gray DB, editors. The reading brain: the biological basis of dyslexia. Parkton (MD): York Press; 1991. p. 53–87.

[18] Meng H, Smith SD, Hager K, et al. DCDC2 is associated with reading disability and modulates neuronal development in the brain. Proc Natl Acad Sci U S A 2005;102(47):17053–8.

[19] Schumacher J, Anthoni H, Dahdouh F, et al. Strong genetic evidence of DCDC2 as a susceptibility gene for dyslexia. Am J Hum Genet 2006;78(1).

[20] Cope N, Harold D, Hill G, et al. Strong evidence that KIAA0319 on chromosome 6p is a susceptibility gene for developmental dyslexia. Am J Hum Genet 2005;76(4):581–91 [Epub 2005 Feb 16].

[21] Hannula-Jouppi K, Kaminen-Ahola N, Taipale M, et al. The axon guidance receptor gene ROBO1 is a candidate gene for developmental dyslexia. PLoS Genet 2005;1(4):467–74.

[22] Taipale M, Kaminen N, Nopola-Hemmi J, et al. A candidate gene for developmental dyslexia encodes a nuclear tetratricopeptide repeat domain protein dynamically regulated in brain. Proc Natl Acad Sci U S A 2003;100(20):11553–8.

[23] Fletcher JM, Shaywitz SE, Shankweiler DP, et al. Cognitive profiles of reading disability: comparisons of discrepancy and low achievement definitions. J Educ Psychol 1994;86(1):6–23.

[24] Liberman IY, Shankweiler D. Phonology and beginning to read: a tutorial. In: Rieben L, Perfetti CA, editors. Learning to read: basic research and its implications. Hillsdale (NJ): Lawrence Erlbaum; 1991. p. 3–17.

[25] Shankweiler D, Liberman IY, Mark LS, et al. The speech code and learning to read. J Exp Psychol [Hum Learn] 1979;5(6):531–45.

[26] Torgesen J, Wagner R. Alternative diagnostic approaches for specific developmental reading disabilities. In: Manuscript prepared for the National Research Council's Board on Testing and Assessment. Presented at the workshop on IQ Testing and Educational Decision Making; May 11, 1995; Washington, DC; 1995.

[27] Wagner R, Torgesen J. The nature of phonological processes and its causal role in the acquisition of reading skills. Psychol Bull 1987;101:192–212.

[28] Stanovich KE, Siegel LS. Phenotypic performance profile of children with reading disabilities: a regression-based test of the phonological-core variable-difference model. J Educ Psychol 1994;86(1):24–53.

[29] Shaywitz S, Fletcher J, Holahan J, et al. Persistence of dyslexia: the Connecticut Longitudinal Study at adolescence. Pediatrics 1999;104(6):1351–9.

[30] Morris RD, Stuebing KK, Fletcher JM, et al. Subtypes of reading disability: variability around a phonological core. J Educ Psychol 1998;90:347–73.

[31] Ramus F, Rosen S, Dakin S, et al. Theories of developmental dyslexia: insights from a multiple case study of dyslexic adults. Brain 2003;126:841–65.

[32] Report of the National Reading Panel. Teaching children to read: an evidence based assessment of the scientific research literature on reading and its implications for reading instruction: U.S. Department of Health and Human Services, Public Health Service, National Institutes of Health, National Institute of Child Health and Human Development; 2000.

[33] Dejerine J. Sur un cas de cécité verbale avec agraphie, suivi d'autopsie. C.R. Société du Biologie 1891;43:197–201 [in French].

[34] Anderson A, Gore J. The physical basis of neuroimaging techniques. Child Adolesc Psychiatric Clin N Am 1997;6:213–64.

[35] Frackowiak R, Friston K, Frith C, et al. Human brain function. 2nd edition. San Diego (CA): Academic Press, Elsevier Science; 2004.

[36] Jezzard P, Matthews P, Smith S, et al. An introduction to methods. Oxford (UK): Oxford University Press; 2001.

[37] Shaywitz S, Shaywitz B, Pugh K, et al. Functional disruption in the organization of the brain for reading in dyslexia. Proc Natl Acad Sci USA 1998;95:2636–41.

[38] Shaywitz B, Shaywitz S, Pugh K, et al. Disruption of posterior brain systems for reading in children with developmental dyslexia. Biol Psychiatry 2002;52(2):101–10.

[39] Price C, Mechelli A. Reading and reading disturbance. Curr Opin Neurobiol 2005;15:231–8.

[40] Fiez JA, Peterson SE. Neuroimaging studies of word reading. Proc Natl Acad Sci U S A 1998;95(3):914–21.

[41] Logan G. Toward an instance theory of automatization. Psychol Rev 1988;95:492–527.

[42] Logan G. Automaticity and reading: perspectives from the instance theory of automatization. Reading and Writing Quarterly: Overcoming Learning Disabilities 1997;13:123–46.

[43] McCandliss B, Cohen L, Dehaene S. The visual word form area: expertise in reading in the fusiform gyrus. Trends Cogn Sci 2003;7(7):293–9.

[44] Cohen L, Jobert A, Le Bihan D, et al. Distinct unimodal and multimodal regions for word processing in the left temporal cortex. Neuroimage 2004,23(4):1256–70.

[45] Dehaene S, Cohen L, Sigman M, et al. The neural code for written words: a proposal. Trends Cogn Sci 2005;9(7):335–41.

[46] Nakamura K, Dehaene S, Jobert A, et al. Subliminal convergence of kanji and kana words: further evidence for functional parcellation of the posterior temporal cortex in visual word perception. Journal of Cognitive Neuroscience 2005;17(6):954–68.

[47] McCrory E, Mechelli A, Frith U, et al. More than words: a common neural basis for reading and naming deficits in developmental dyslexia? Brain 2005;128(2):261–7.

[48] Shaywitz B, Shaywitz S, Blachman B, et al. Development of left occipito-temporal systems for skilled reading in children after a phonologically-based intervention. Biol Psychiatry 2004;55:926–33.

[49] Wagner RK, Torgesen JK, Rashotte CA. CTOPP examiner's manual. Austin (TX): PRO-ED, Inc.; 1999.

[50] Mather N, Woodcock RW. Woodcock-Johnson III tests of achievement—examiner's manual standard and extended batteries. Itasca (IL): Riverside Publishing; 2001.

[51] Woodcock RW. Woodcock reading mastery tests—revised/normative update (WRMT-R/NU). Bloomington (MN): Pearson Assessments; 1987.

[52] Wiederholt JL, Bryant BR. GORT-4 examiner's manual. Austin (TX): PRO-ED, Inc.; 2001.

[53] Torgesen JK, Wagner RK, Rashotte CA. TOWRE examiner's manual. Austin (TX): PRO-ED, Inc.; 1999.

[54] Wilkinson G. Wide range achievement test-3. Austin (TX): PRO-ED, Inc.; 1994.

[55] Larsen SC, Hammill ED, Moats LC. Test of written spelling-4. San Antonio (TX): Psychological Corporation; 1999.

[56] Brown JI, Fishco VV, Hanna GS. Nelson Denny reading test—manual for scoring and iInterpretation (forms G and H). Itasca (IL): Riverside Publishing; 1993.

[57] Ben-Dror I, Pollatsek A, Scarpati A. Word identification in isolation and in context by college dyslexic students. Brain Lang 1991;40:471–90.

[58] Bruck M. Outcomes of adults with childhood histories of dyslexia. In: Hulme C, Joshi R, editors. Reading and spelling: development and disorders. Mahwah (NJ): Lawrence Erlbaum Associates; 1998. p. 179–200.

[59] Lefly DL, Pennington BF. Spelling errors and reading fluency in compensated adult dyslexics. Ann Dyslexia 1991;41:143–62.

[60] Torgesen J, Wagner R, Rashotte C, et al. Preventing reading failure in young children with phonological processing disabilities. J Educ Psychol 1999;91:579–93.

[61] Foorman BR, Brier JI, Fletcher JM. Interventions aimed at improving reading success: an evidence-based approach. Dev Neuropsychol 2003;24:613–39.

ELSEVIER
SAUNDERS

PEDIATRIC CLINICS

OF NORTH AMERICA

Pediatr Clin N Am 54 (2007) 625–642

Early Literacy Interventions: Reach Out and Read

Earnestine Willis, MD, MPH[a,*],
Claudia Kabler-Babbitt[a],
Barry Zuckerman, MD[b]

[a]Department of Pediatrics, Medical College of Wisconsin, 8701 Watertown Plank Road,
Milwaukee, WI 53226, USA
[b]Department of Pediatrics, Boston City Hospital, 818 Harrison Avenue, Boston,
MA 02118–2999, USA

The linked cycles of illiteracy and poverty are well documented and they have a major impact on a child's early literacy development and future school performance. Children's earliest literacy encounters occur in their homes with families. Literacy has been defined as using printed and written information to function in society, to achieve one's goals, and to develop one's knowledge and potential [1]. Early literacy, or preliteracy, has been defined as a child's literacy-related exposures and experiences from birth until solo reading. Examples of early literacy behaviors are knowledge of book handling, looking at and recognizing pictures in books, picture and story comprehension, reading imitative behaviors, memorizing and repeating rhymes or story refrains, and making up their own stories [2]. Health literacy has been defined as the degree to which individuals have the capacity to obtain, process, and understand basic health information and services needed to make appropriate health decisions [3]. Levels of literacy have also been defined: (1) basic literacy consists of having skills to perform simple and everyday literacy activities, (2) intermediate literacy consists of having skills to perform moderately challenging literacy activities, and (3) proficient literacy consists of having the skills to perform more complex and challenging literacy activities. For example, below basic literacy includes adults who have the ability to read short text, locate a piece of information based on a literal match, and perform single, simple arithmetic. Throughout this article it is important to refer back to these definitions as early literacy intervention is discussed [4,5].

* Corresponding author.
E-mail address: ewillis@mcw.edu (E. Willis).

0031-3955/07/$ - see front matter © 2007 Elsevier Inc. All rights reserved.
doi:10.1016/j.pcl.2007.02.012
pediatric.theclinics.com

Shared literacy experiences include not only book-sharing with each child, but also singing, telling stories and jokes, object naming, and casual talking. A child's range, type, and style of literacy exposures are related to the parent's level of literacy, personal early literacy experiences, education, employment, available resources, domestic situations, and other factors. This section considers some of the demographics of literacy level and poverty in the United States and summarizes the association of family literacy activities with a child's literacy development. In addition, early language development is reviewed, and how the home literacy environment contributes to literacy development is described. The American Academy of Pediatrics has acknowledged the Reach Out and Read (ROR) model as a standard of care for early literacy promotion and endorses its incorporation into every pediatrician's practice. Finally, the lessons learned from early literacy interventions are described: ROR, as an intervention in language development, and how primary care providers for children can support children's literacy development during routine care encounters with each child and their families.

Literacy in low-income children

Nearly half of all Americans were functioning at below basic or marginal literacy level in 1992 [6]. A follow-up survey by the National Assessment of Adult Literacy 10 years later revealed that 53% of adults had intermediate health literacy, 22% had basic health literacy, and 14% had below basic health literacy. Disproportionally, large numbers of those with poor literacy skills come from low-income backgrounds, and 43% of those with the lowest literacy skills live in poverty [7,8]. In 2004, 37 million people were living in poverty, an increase of 1.1 million from the previous year [9]. The low literacy levels of the nation's children do not seem to be improving and the risk of low literacy threatens an ever larger portion of this nation's children. Since 1992, the average literacy achievement for high-performing students has improved, whereas the average for low-performing students has dropped [10]. In 2005, according to the National Association of Educational Progress, 29% of eighth graders and 38% of fourth graders scored below basic reading levels. Children are at risk for low literacy when their parents' literacy skills are poor, or a limited or poor quality education. According to Raikes and colleagues [11], the odds that mothers read out loud on a daily basis to their preschool children were increased by each year of the mothers' education. In 2004, 16% of United States children lived in a family where the head of the household was a high school dropout. In the same year, 19% of children spoke a language other than English at home, which adds another confounder in estimating literacy levels, because the parent may be literate in their native language [12]. Literacy level and school achievement have enormous economic consequences; having high school skill levels doubles the probability of employment, and high school graduates earn 42% more than those with less education [13–15].

The Carnegie Starting Points report of 1994 noted that one in three children enter kindergarten unprepared to learn and lacking language skills that are the prerequisite of literacy acquisition. The children at greatest risk for poor literacy outcomes are disproportionately from low-income populations. Factors contributing to the risk of poor literacy skills are absence or scarcity of reading materials in the home, economic insecurity, lack of educational processes in the home, poor parent-child interactions, intergenerational beliefs, attitude and behaviors, parental attitudes toward education and emergent literacy, and deficiencies in the school systems [16]. Just as African Americans and Latinos are more likely to live in low-income families, they are also more likely to have lower literacy skills. School dropouts are more common among African Americans, Latinos, and immigrant populations. At least 75% of today's jobs require at least a ninth grade reading level, and employment is an essential path to economic security [8].

Low literacy contributes to unemployment, crime, poverty, welfare dependency, and poor health status. Although inadequate literacy pervades society, so too does inadequate health literacy. Studies show, for example, that the reading skills of patients with asthma must be considered when providing care and health education [17,18]. Williams and coworkers [18] demonstrated that a patient's literacy skills are a strong predictor of asthma knowledge and metered-dose inhaler technique. Another current and important example is found in evolving HIV-AIDS treatment regimens. People with poor reading skills are less likely to access and comprehend the rapidly changing information about HIV-AIDS treatments, thereby decreasing care and compliance and increasing morbidity and mortality [19]. Lower literacy patients are more dependent on providers for information and may require more visits, longer visits, and communications tailored to manage appropriately their health. Providers need to be cognizant of misinterpretation of health and treatment information and behaviors that might not be consistent with scientifically supported HIV treatment and prevention methods [19]. It is essential to understand the significant role that inadequate literacy plays in the management of chronic health conditions that affect children and adolescents, such as hypertension, diabetes, HIV/AIDS, and asthma. Researchers need to examine the roles of literacy more thoroughly in low-income and racial–ethnic groups for preventable and controllable health conditions.

Many children living in impoverished communities have lower reading levels compared with children living in more affluent communities. Morrow [20] reported that children who entered school with little experience with books and reading became poorer readers than children with richer experiences. The number and variety of age-appropriate books in a child's home varies considerably. Young children are dependent on parents and caregivers for access to books, and for the quality and quantity of their book interactions. In the study by Raikes and coworkers [11], most of the young children had access to at least a few books; by age 2, 85% of the children had five or more children's books. Another study paints a grimmer picture; almost one in four low-income children has less than 10 books of any kind in his or her home [21]. The caregiver's culture, childhood reading experiences, verbal ability, education, and warmth affect the level of engagement between the child and parent, as well as the quality and style of reading.

Morrow [20] also found that having a library card being taken to the library often, and being read to regularly were related to a child's early interest in reading and ability to read early. Raikes and coworkers [11] recognized that there are multiple barriers to library usage. Some of these barriers are living in outlying rural areas or unsafe urban neighborhoods, or being without reliable, affordable transportation. Families may simply have no time available to travel to and spend at the library, apart from the daily struggle to survive. Books borrowed from the library must also be returned, requiring a second trip, and if the trip is not made on time, fines may be incurred. Compared with 40% of families with incomes above the poverty threshold, only 24% of low-income families visited the library [22]. It has been recognized for several decades that children begin the process of learning to read long before they enter formal schooling [23,24]. In addition, such activities as storytelling, finger plays, and singing songs encourages the acquisition of literacy skills [25,26]. A growing number of children live in households where the language spoken in school settings is not the same as the language that students hear spoken at home. Children living in poverty tend disproportionately to attend schools with limited resources and may be at risk by virtue of crowded classrooms, overstressed teachers, and poor reading support. The education they receive does not put them on a trajectory to break free of their disadvantaged backgrounds. In the nation's highest poverty public schools, an amazing 68% of fourth graders fail to reach the basic reading level. Only about 1 in 10 of the fourth graders at many of these schools can read at the expected proficient level [27]. Their educational settings are characterized by high-stress teaching and learning environments, by overcrowding, poor-quality facilities, and depleted libraries. The schools are staffed with fewer qualified librarians and fewer well-qualified teachers, and may have teachers and administrators who have low expectations of the students [28].

McQuillan [28] made the case that lack of reading time and the lack of access to reading materials are fundamental barriers to reading success. A typical middle-class child enters the first grade with 1000 to 1700 cumulative hours of one-on-one picture book reading, whereas a child from a low-income family averages just 25 hours [29,30]. A child from a low-income family enters kindergarten with a listening vocabulary of 3000 words, whereas a child from a middle-income family enters kindergarten with a listening vocabulary of 20,000 words [31]. It is evident that poverty and poor literacy acquisition cross in a variety of ways to put low-income children at real risk for greater health and economic vulnerability.

Sixteen percent of parents of children 3 years old or younger do not read with their children and 23% do so only once or twice a week [32]. More recent findings estimate that only 50% of low-income mothers of children 3 years old or younger read daily to their children. Interestingly, as a child reaches 14 months, the child's chances of daily reading increase significantly if the child is female or a firstborn. For older children, 24 to 36 months old, these "odds increased by maternal verbal ability or education level as well as by the child being firstborn or participating in Early Head Start." The data analysis suggests the reciprocal and snowballing relationship between mother and child book sharing and her children's vocabulary [11].

Home literacy profile

It has been accepted that the home literacy environment influences a child's literacy development. What children experience before they begin formal schooling affects where they land on the continuum of school readiness and should be considered a significant source of influence in literacy development [31]. Griffin and Morrison [33] assessed the influence of home literacy environment using questions to define home literacy environment. These questions included presence or absence of reading materials in the home (newspapers, child and adult magazines, and children books); frequency of library visits; frequency of observable literacy-related behaviors (mother and father reading to themselves); frequency with which an adult reads to the child; and the frequency of one literacy-competitive behavior (television viewing) [33]. After controlling for the effect of parents' intelligence quotient and social background, they found that a child having a richer home literacy environment is associated with higher language-based literacy, specifically receptive vocabulary, general knowledge, and reading recognition skills during kindergarten. These findings were not associated with number-based literacy and other constellation of factors that might influence number-based literacy, such as frequency of playing counting games and number of math workbooks, might yield stronger math skills. He also found that the effects of home literacy environments on language-based literacy persisted through the end of second grade. Other researchers have shown that other aspects of the home environment, such as reading and storytelling, stimulates the imagination; fosters the development of children's vocabulary; and introduces them to components of stories, such as character, plot, action, and sequence [34,35]. Many families are actively involved in helping their young children learn. There are differences, however, in families' type and style of engagement in literacy activities according to the families' race and ethnicity. Latino and African American children were less likely than white children to have been read to, told stories to, or participated in arts and crafts with their families three or more times in the last week. This is consistent with the findings of Raikes and colleagues [11] that even low-income white mothers read with their children more often than Latino or African American mothers.

A number of risk factors are believed to have an impact on the development of literacy skills. These risk factors include a mother with less than a high school education, living with fewer than two parents, living in a family with an income below the poverty threshold, living in a home whose parents speak a language other than English, and having a race or ethnicity other than white. For example, a study conducted by the US Department of Education's National Center for Education Statistics 1999 reported that 70% of children living in families with incomes below the poverty threshold were read to three or more times in the last week, compared with 85% of children living above the poverty threshold. Children with two or more risk factors are less likely than other children to show signs of emerging literacy. Children who are read to frequently are almost twice as likely as other children to show three or more skills associated with emerging literacy. Children who were told stories, taught letters, words, or numbers three or more times in the previous week, or visited the library in the previous month were more likely than other children to show signs of emerging literacy. Daily reading can even be used as a predictor for a child's language and cognition level at 36 months [11].

Language development and reading

The development of phonologic sensitivity and letter knowledge starts in infancy, a time when neuronal synaptic proliferation can be influenced by a child's experiences and exposures. Language interventions that build vocabulary and decontextualized language structures need to occur before instruction on how to decode written words, rather than later. Language development is fundamental to emergent literacy. Snow and Tabors [36] indicate that being read to early and often supports the development of a foundation for later learning and ultimate reading success. Shore [37] reveals that reading aloud to infants stimulates their brains to create new learning pathways and strengthens existing ones. Interactions with caregivers mold brain development and foster neural reorganization from phonologic development in the first year of life, followed by a burst of semantic and syntactic development during the second and third years, respectively. During the early childhood years, children acquire skills with the social uses of languages (pragmatics or communication skills). Some researchers suggest that emergent literacy consist of six child characteristics to be emphasized and balanced in literacy development: (1) oral language, (2) phonologic sensitivity, (3) letter knowledge, (4) print awareness, (5) print motivation, and (6) emergent reading and writing [25]. Young children's vocabulary has an impact on decoding skills very early in the process of learning to read, but the mechanism to explain this relationship is unknown. The recognition of increased segmentation of words supports the acquisition of higher levels of phonologic sensitivity. First, young children detect similar and dissimilar sounding words; next, they blend words together and then learn to remove sounds from words. The ability to substitute sounds is learned later in a child's development. As linguistic complexity develops, phonologic sensitivity begins to manifest as an awareness of phonemes, with the precise timing greatly dependent on instructional experiences in phonologic sensitivity or letter knowledge. More specifically, activities designed to foster phonologic sensitivity of prereaders, like blending syllables, ease the learning of higher levels of phonologic sensitivity, like deleting phonemes, which is known to play a casual role in reading acquisition [25].

Children generally learn the names of letters before they learn the sounds that correspond to those letters. Learning the names of letters, however, does not have a direct effect on learning to read [29]. It may be that having some knowledge of letters is required before higher levels of phonologic sensitivity, such as phonemic awareness, can be learned. Reading follows a number of print concepts, such as progressing from the front to the end of a book, page by page, from left to right, and reading words from left to right and top to bottom on a page. Knowledge of these print concepts is correlated with emergent literacy skills.

Young and colleagues [32] documented the child-rearing concerns of parents and the parents' health care experiences in a national survey about children from birth to 3 years of age. Only 39% of the parents reported regular involvement in reading or looking at a book with their children more than once a day. Approximately one third of the parents reported playing with their children each day, or singing or playing music more than once a day with their child. Parents also indicated that if pediatricians encouraged breast-feeding or reading more frequently for their children, the encouragement would influence parents' behaviors. Pediatricians should be more engaged in supporting parenting skills that help children to learn, and these include early reading and use of music to promote active brain development, motivation, and child self-esteem in families [32]. Once children are physically capable of affecting their own literacy environment, emergent literacy advocates have suggested that children's interest in literacy activities plays a crucial role in reading acquisition. Thomas [38] found that early readers play with, enjoy, and value reading readiness toys, such as books and alphabet cards, more than young nonreaders. Many researchers have advocated that shared reading promotes oral language development. The following findings have supported that position:

- Vocabulary learning from listening to stories is predicted by the frequency of the word in the text, depiction of words in illustrations, and the amount of redundancy of the word in the text [39].
- Multiple readings of storybooks enhance expressive and receptive vocabulary acquisition [40].
- Storybook reading positively impacts vocabulary when concrete objects are used to represent the words; children have multiple opportunities to

use the book-related words, involvement of children in conversation, and activities about the stories [41].
• Using techniques of dialogic reading, through which the child learns to become the storyteller [42].

Foorman and colleagues [43] argue that oral language development is a superordinate component of emergent literacy and that differences in children's vocabulary size most frequently occur when English is being learned as a second language or because of limited learning opportunities in the home. Experts consider that assessment of phonologic awareness skills and Diagnostic Evaluation of Language Variations Screening Test are useful tools for determining language development.

Reach Out and Read model

ROR was established for the benefit of children and families by pediatricians and educators in Boston as a nationwide early literacy intervention. This nonprofit program is endorsed by the American Academy of Pediatrics. The mission of ROR is to make literacy promotion a standard part of pediatric primary care, so that children grow up with books and a love for reading. Since 1989, ROR has grown to more than 2948 hospitals and health centers (44% of sites are in urban areas, 20% in rural areas, 13% in suburban areas, and 23% not identified) throughout the United States, Guam, and Puerto Rico, serving more than 2.5 million children each year. Annually, more than 4.1 million new books are given to children and 44,100 physicians and nurses have been trained in the ROR strategies in early literacy guidance. Sixty-seven percent of ROR providers report that they are able to give literacy guidance and books during at least 80% of health supervision visits. ROR is responsive to multicultural and immigrant families, and makes books available in 12 different languages. In 2004, the US Department of Education provided ROR $4 million to buy books; this was increased to $10 million for 2005. Needlman reported [44] that parents who were encouraged by their pediatricians to read to their child and given books were four times more likely to report loving to read aloud to their children. By participating in ROR, each child is potentially given 10 books, raising their book ownership above the level seen in most low-income families.

Routinely, the ROR model consists of the following components:

Health care providers (pediatricians, nurses, residents, nurse practitioners, physician assistants, and family practitioners) are trained in techniques to promote the parents' early literacy efforts with their children. This anticipatory guidance is incorporated into every well-child visit from 6 months to 5 years.

As part of these well-child checks (6 months–5 years), health care providers give each child a developmental and culturally appropriate new book to take home to enrich the home-literacy environment, especially important for low-income families.

During the health check visit (children ages 6 months–5 years), medical providers incorporate the new book into the developmental assessment to observe the child's interest, early literacy, or emergent literacy skills and their fine motor abilities.

Volunteer readers are located in the waiting rooms of the clinical setting, providing literacy experiences for the children and modeling reading aloud for parents. Parents learn to be more flexible when reading and to maximize interactive and dialogic reading. They can also find that very young children enjoy looking at picture books and older children enjoy storytelling interactions with adult caregivers.

Pediatricians support use of the library as children develop an interest in books, and when indicated, adult literacy referrals for parents who have family literacy concerns.

Although each ROR program has unique components, such as literacy partners and set up of "ROR literacy corners" located in the waiting room, they are all versions of the ROR national model. For example, ROR-Milwaukee was initiated in October 1997 and co-sponsored by Children's Hospital and Health System and the Medical College of Wisconsin. ROR-Milwaukee programs are located in predominantly low-income sites (two federally qualified health centers and an outpatient setting for training residents in general pediatrics). Other ROR-Milwaukee program partners include college students from the Service Learning Programs of two higher education institutions, senior citizens affiliation, and community members as volunteer readers in the waiting rooms. Local bookstore vendors and community organizations donate new and gently used books for older siblings of ROR participants. Another model might have book distribution in migrant health centers or with police officers as partners.

These combined efforts contribute to the development of the emergent literacy skills needed as precursors to formal reading and to long-term successful school performance. Families served by ROR programs learn that children should be read to at a very early age. Other researchers have demonstrated that early regular experience with book reading, beginning as young as 14 months, is particularly beneficial [45,46]. Programs are usually operated through an interdisciplinary team with the ROR medical director conducting provider training, and the ROR program coordinator monitoring the program quality, funding, and book donations to the program. In many states, the executive director of the American Academy of Pediatrics has become engaged in the dissemination of the program into pediatrician practices and frequently acts as the fiscal agent for ROR grant funds. Most states have local foundations and corporations funding their early literacy interventions, with the national ROR supporting at least 25% of the funds to purchase books for low-income families.

Impact of Reach Out and Read

Repeated studies have demonstrated the benefits of early reading to children. Review of the scientific literature demonstrates that ROR is an evidence-based intervention in language development and the home literacy environment. Some of these benefits include increased language development, higher standardized vocabulary scores for receptive and expressive language, positive changes in attitudes about reading, and a contribution to a positive home literacy environment. Literacy is a continuous developmental process that includes listening, speaking, reading, and writing. In 1985, the National Commission on Reading reported that reading aloud to children is the single most important activity for literacy development and eventual reading success. ROR encourages pediatricians (and other child health care providers) to guide parents to start book-related activities (with a developmentally appropriate book) with their children as early as 6 months of age and to promote reading by modeling reading in waiting rooms.

High and colleagues [47] evaluated the effectiveness of a literacy intervention delivered by pediatric providers as a part of well-child care on parental attitudes and behaviors and on child language. A multicultural group of low-income families were randomized to an intervention group and control group. Families in the intervention group were given developmentally appropriate books and educational materials, and counseled to share books frequently with their children, whereas the control group was not given any of those interventions. Using the MacArthur Communication and Development Inventory and the Child-Centered Literacy Orientation at the time of enrollment and again 9 to 12 months later, an increase in literacy-related activities in the intervention group was observed. This study also showed that parents changed their attitudes about the importance of reading with their infants and toddlers, and expressing an enjoyment of reading together. The receptive and expressive vocabulary scores were higher in the intervention group, especially for the older toddlers [47]. Twelve other studies published in peer-reviewed scientific journals have showed that ROR is effective in promoting reading aloud and language development in children. These studies can be summarized as follows:

> Needlman's and coworkers [44] study showed that parents given books and guidance were four times more likely to report loving to read aloud or doing it in the previous 24 hours. This association increased to approximately eight times more likely to report loving to read aloud for children on Aid to Families with Dependent Children.
> Snow and Tabors [36] demonstrated that being read to early and often furthers a strong foundation for learning and successful reading skill development.
> Sanders and colleagues [48] conducted a study that suggested that ROR programs increase parent-child book sharing within Latino immigrant

families, even when a single book is given, and that parents quickly became advocates for their young children's emergent literacy.

Jones and colleagues [49] studied the comparison of anticipatory guidance to promote early literacy at well-child care visits with and without giving a book. The study reveals that parents were twice as receptive to their physicians' helpfulness and to engage their children in literacy activities as the families receiving only anticipatory guidance.

In a similar randomized control intervention study of Latino families, Latino families receiving children's books from a pediatrician were three times more likely to report book sharing as one of the three favorite activities that they do with their children [50].

Mendelsohn and coworkers [51] compared a ROR clinic and a similar non-ROR clinic and the former clinic evidenced significantly higher scores on standardized vocabulary tests for receptive and expressive language. A similar study by Sharif and coworkers [52] confirmed these results.

Weitzman and coworkers [53] demonstrated that for children ages 18 to 30 months, ROR contributes positively to a child's home literacy environment, after an interview in the clinical waiting room followed by home observation measurements of the literacy environment.

Flexible approaches across developmental levels (Table 1) provide suggestions for incorporating reading into developmental and behavioral assessments of the children and parent-child interactions. Associations between family literacy activities and children's emerging literacy were reported by Lonigan and colleagues [54], who found that the print motivation of 2 year olds was closely related to the age that the children were first read to by their parents. They suggested that children having greater experiences with shared reading display more interest in literacy-related activities [46,54]. Other studies have supported the role of intervention programs, such as Early Head Start, that influence the literacy experiences parents provide children and the promotion of early language development [55–58].

Discussion and recommendations

Engaging children in early literacy activities that enrich parent-child interactions can play an essential role in emergent literacy skills, helping children to be prepared for school. Early literacy begins in a child's first days with caring connections between parents and babies. These contacts include talking, singing, telling stories, book reading, rhyming, object naming, word games, and other family events. The greater the number and variety of these connections, including the child's access to books, the greater the likelihood of the child's school success.

Table 1
Literacy books and guidance for parents based on developmental milestones

Ages	Developmental milestones	Behaviors	Recommended books	Guidance to parents
6–12 mo	Able to grasp Hand to mouth activities. Able to sit up, crawl. Comprehends words. Babbles.	Attentive to vocal intonations. Visually tracks fallen objects. Inspects objects, then mouths, then bangs. Excited by picture book, grabs, mouths Plays peek-a-boo, pat-a-cake.	Board or cloth books with limited text and colorful pictures. Enjoys pictures of baby faces, books with one image per page.	Incorporate books/stories/singing into bedtime routine. Interest may be very brief, 5–15 min.
13–24 mo	Explores world through walking and climbing. Begins talking, using short phrases. Points to desired objects with finger, labeling.	Able to be consoled. Explores away from parents lap Reads' parents' expressions. Looks for hidden object, in play, Uses objects correctly. Works wind up toys, on-off buttons Points with finger at images on pages.	Board books with bright pictures and some words, with minimal plots. Enjoys silly stories, books featuring objects from their everyday life, children, food, animals. Able to point at book images, hold book, turn book right side up.	Select reading aloud time for pleasure and when child is ready. Let child select and control book. Ask child questions about book. Let child complete sentences when reading. Child may request the same book to be read repeatedly. Attention span longer, but variable may be up to 20 min.
25–35 mo	Able to go up and down steps independently. Speaking many words and simple sentences Begins naming body parts. Able to hold crayon Able to copy "O."	Very active and assertive about preferences. May be clingy In play, understands one thing stands for another. (substitution) Combines play actions (rocks doll, puts to bed).	Board books still best, books with flaps or other interactive devices help hold attention. Loves to learn new things, new animals, new objects, colors. Able to understand that the images relate to the words read and that the markings on the page indicate what words to be read. May "read" familiar books to self or to others.	Continue bedtime reading routine. Child enjoys turning pages, holding the book. Read interactively, using dialogical technique. Attention span varies, 5–30 min.

Age				
3–5 y	Able to jump with both feet off floor, balance on one foot briefly. Speaking in longer sentences, mostly correct use of grammar, asks questions. Can copy +, stick figure, later can copy a square or triangle.	Plays out familiar events, changes outcomes. Talks for dolls, assigns roles to other children, imaginary scripts. Plays well with group of children. Understands taking turns, uses words not hitting.	Paperback books and more complex stories, about friends and families. Books with intricate illustrations that capture their attention while the text is being read. Can move finger along with text being read. Beginning to learn to write letters, their name. Understands that text is read right to left and top to bottom on pages.	Continue to make reading an interactive experience, let child tell parents the story. Able to anticipate "what happens next" in stories. Attention span ranges up to 40 min.

Data from **ROR** Developmental Milestones of Early Literacy and **ROR** Medical Provider Developmental Code Card.

Pediatricians are uniquely positioned to address a child's literacy development and foster positive parenting because they are often the only practitioner regularly encountering parents, infants, and children during the preschool years. ROR has been designed to target low-income families by providing materials, education, and support to focus on books and reading aloud as one of the most important parenting skills in parent-child interaction. Promoting literacy development begins with an assessment of the targeted child and the parent for reading experience. Health care providers must be aware of the potential barriers that interfere with parent–child literacy activities. These barriers include limited parent education, parent language and the family's social characteristics, such as busy work schedule, parental literacy level and attitudes about reading, substance abuse, mental health issues, family violence, and so forth as nonsupportive factors to literacy encouragement during childhood. Literacy activities should be pleasurable and strategically tailored to the needs and developmental level of the parents and child, respectively [51]. Language and cultural diversity are becoming more important as the population of the United States changes. For example, "Parents of young children with limited English proficiency may need extra encouragement to engage in some of these activities. Many times parents' language skills may be limited, or they may hesitate to use their native language at home, assuming that it will not help their children succeed in school. Some parents whose culture emphasizes speaking to children in a directive style may benefit from coaching to try a more conversational style. This practice gives parents another way to nurture their child's language skills and vocabulary development" [59]. "Some parents who don't speak English are less likely to expose their children to early literacy experiences than English-speaking parents" [60]. "In general, mothers whose first language is not English are less likely to read to their children regularly" [61]. Some of these parents may believe that it is the role of the schools to address literacy for their child [62].

Many low-income parents face difficult logistical barriers that make time and energy scarce for book reading, library visits, and early language development. This combination of factors can cause many children from low-income homes and homes with limited English proficiency to enter kindergarten behind their peers in language and literacy skills [62]. In addition, having books available in bilingual languages and culturally sensitive to the population are essential [63]. Most of the research presented so far has been based on mother's reports, with very few studies to substantiate the mother's report of literacy activities. One such study by Weitzman and coworkers [53] demonstrated that ROR contributed a small but significant influence on child's home literacy profile by home assessments. More research is necessary to determine if the parent-child home literacy activities can be significantly influenced by activities recommended or modeled within practices. Several studies, however, have shown a positive relationship between literacy promotion and parent-child interactions and child language development. Although the authors believe that these early literacy building blocks support stronger performance on reading comprehension when entering school, there is still a need to conduct longitudinal studies to support these correlations objectively.

Acknowledgments

The authors thank Teri Wermager for her diligent assistance in the development and organization of this manuscript, and Dr. Perri Klass for her thoughtful review, edits, and comments.

References

[1] Kaestle CF, Campbell A, Finn JD, et al. Adult literacy and education in America: four studies based on the national adult literacy survey. Washington, DC: U.S. Department of Education, National Center for Education Statistics; 1999.

[2] Boston University Medical Center, Erikson Institute and Zero to Three. Early literacy. Available at: www.zerotothree.org/BrainWonders. Accessed October 13, 2006.

[3] Institute of Medicine. Health literacy: a prescription to end confusion. Washington, DC: Institute of Medicine, Board on Neuroscience and Behavioral Health, Committee on Health Literacy; 2004.

[4] White S, Dillow S. Key concepts and features of the 2003 national assessment of adult literacy. Washington, DC: U.S. Government Printing Office: U.S. Department of Education, National Center for Education Statistics; 2005. NCES 2006–471.

[5] Institute of Medicine. Measuring literacy: performance levels for adults, interim report. Washington, DC: National Academies Press; 2005.

[6] Kirsch IS, Jungeblut A, Jenkins L, et al. Adult literacy in America. Washington DC: National Center for Education Statistics; 1993.

[7] Fotheringham JB, Creal D. Family socioeconomic and educational emotional characteristics as predictors of school achievement. J Educ Res 1980;73:311–7.

[8] National Institute for Literacy. Fast facts on literacy. Washington, DC: National Institute for Literacy; 1998.

[9] DeNavas-Walt C, Proctor BD, Lee CL. Income, poverty and health insurance coverage in the United States: 2004. Washington, DC: U.S. Government Printing Office; 2005. p. 60–229.

[10] National Center for Education Statistics - The National Assessment of Educational Progress. Reading gap widens between high - and low-performing fourth-grade students. Available at: http://nces.ed.gov/Pressrelease/rel2001/4_6_01.asp. Accessed September 8, 2006.

[11] Raikes H, Luze G, Brooks-Gunn J, et al. Mother-child bookreading in low-income families: correlates and outcomes during the first three years of life. Child Dev 2006;77:924–53.

[12] US Census Bureau. American community survey, 2004. Language Spoken at Home (S1601) and Selected Characteristics of People at Specified Levels of Poverty in the Past 12 Months (S1703).

[13] ProLiteracy America. U.S. adult literacy programs: making a difference. A review of research on positive outcomes achieved by literacy programs and the people they serve. Syracuse (NY): US Programs Division of ProLiteracy Worldwide; 2003.

[14] National Institute for Literacy. National literacy summit foundation paper. Washington, DC: Institute for Literacy; 2000.

[15] Carnevale A, Desrochers D. The missing middle: aligning education and the knowledge economy. Paper presented at "Preparing America's Future: the High School Symposium"

sponsored by the Office of Vocational Education, U.S. Dept. of Education. Washington, DC, April 4, 2002.

[16] Cronan TA, Cruz SG, Arriaga RI. The effects of a community-based literacy program on young children's language and conceptual development. Am J Community Psychol 1996;24:251–72.

[17] Lang DM, Sherman MS, Polansky M. Guidelines and realities of asthma management: the Philadelphia story. Arch Intern Med 1997;157:1193–200.

[18] Williams M, Baker DW, Honig EG, et al. Inadequate literacy is a barrier to asthma knowledge and self-care. Chest 1998;11:1008–15.

[19] Kalichman SE, Benotsch E, Saurez T, et al. Health literacy and health-related knowledge among persons living with HIV/AIDS. Am J Prev Med 2000;18:325–31.

[20] Morrow LM. Home and school correlates of early interest in literature. J Educ Res 1983;76: 221–30.

[21] High PC, Hopmann M, LaGrasse L, et al. Child centered literacy orientation: a form of social capital? Pediatrics 1999;103:e55.

[22] National Center for Education Statistics (NCES). National household education survey. Washington, DC: U.S. Department of Education; 1999.

[23] Sommenschein S, Brody G, Munsterman K. The influence of family beliefs and practices on children's early reading development. In: Baker P, Afferbach P, Reinking D, editors. Developing engaged readers in school and home communities. Mahwah (NJ): Lawrence Erlbaum Associates; 1996. p. 3–20.

[24] Teale WH, Sulzby E. Emergent literacy: new perspectives. In: Strickland DS, Morrow LM, editors. Emerging literacy: young children learn to read and write. Newark (DE): International Reading Association; 1989. p. 1–9.

[25] Whitehurst GJ, Lonigan CJ. Child development and emergent literacy. Child Dev 1998;69: 848–72.

[26] Whitehurst GJ, Epstein J, Angell A, et al. Outcomes of an emergent literacy intervention in Head Start. J Educ Psychol 1994;86:542–55.

[27] Perie M, Grigg W, Donahue P. The nation's report card: reading 2005. Washington, DC: Government Printing Office: U.S. Department of Education, National Center for Education Statistics; 2005. NCES 2006–451.

[28] McQuillan J. The literacy crisis; false claims, real solutions. Portsmouth (NH): Heinemann; 1998.

[29] Adams MJ. Research on prereaders. In: Beginning to read. Cambridge (MA): MIT Press; 1990. p. 82–91.

[30] Teale WH. Home background and young children's literacy development. In: Teale WH, Sulzby E, editors. Emergent literacy. Norwood (NJ): Ablex Publishing Corporation; 1986. p. 173–206.

[31] Hart B, Risley TR. Meaningful differences in everyday experience of American children. Baltimore (MD): Paul H. Brookes Publishing; 1995.

[32] Young K, Davis K, Schoen C, et al. Listening to parents; a national survey of parents with young children. Arch Pediatr Adolesc Med 1998;152:255–62.

[33] Griffin E, Morrison FJ. The unique contribution of home literacy environment to differences in early literacy skills. Early Child Dev Care 1997;127–128:233–43.

[34] National Education Goals Panel. National education goals report: building a nation of learners. Washington, DC: U.S. Government Printing Office; 1997.

[35] Moss B, Fawcett G. Bringing the curriculum of the world of the home to the school. Reading & Writing Quarterly: Overcoming Learning Difficulties 1995;11:247–56.

[36] Snow C, Tabors P. Intergenerational transfer of literacy. In: Benjamin LA, Lord J, editors. Family literacy: directions in research and implications for practice. Washington, DC: Office of Educational Research and Improvement, U.S. Department of Education; 1996.

[37] Shore R. Rethinking the brain: new insights into early development. New York: Families & Work Institute; 1997.

[38] Thomas B. Early toy preferences of four-year-old readers and nonreaders. Child Dev 1984; 55:424–30.

[39] Elley WB. Vocabulary acquisition from listening to stories. Reading Research Quarterly 1989;24:174–87.

[40] Senechal M, Cornell EH. Vocabulary acquisition through shared reading experiences. Reading Research Quarterly 1993;28:360–75.

[41] Wasik BA, Bond MA. Beyond the pages of a book: interactive book reading and language development in pre-school classrooms. J Educ Psychol 2001;93:243–50.

[42] Whitehurst GJ, Lonigan CJ. Emergent literacy: development from prereaders to readers. In: Neuman SB, Dickinson DK, editors. Handbook of early literacy research. New York: Guilford Press; 2001. p. 11–29.

[43] Foorman BR, Anthony J, Seals L, et al. Language development and emergent literacy in preschool. Semin Pediatr Neurol 2002;9:173–84.

[44] Needlman R, Fried LE, Morley DS, et al. Clinic-based intervention to promote literacy; a pilot study. Am J Dis Child 1991;145:881–4.

[45] DeBaryshe BD. Maternal belief systems: linchpin in the home reading process. J Appl Dev Psychol 1995;16:1–20.

[46] Scarborough HS, Dobrich W, Hager M. Preschool literacy experiences and later reading achievement. J Learn Disabil 1991;24:508–11.

[47] High PC, LaGasse L, Becker S, et al. Literacy promotion in primary care pediatrics: can we make a difference? Pediatrics 2000;105:927–34.

[48] Sanders LM, Gershon TD, Huffman LC, et al. Prescribing books for immigrant children: a pilot study to promote emergent literacy among the children of Hispanic immigrants. Arch Pediatr Adolesc Med 2000;154:771–7.

[49] Jones VF, Franco SM, Metcalf SC, et al. The value of book distribution in a clinic-based literacy intervention program. Clin Pediatr 2000;39:535–41.

[50] Golova N, Alario AJ, Viver PM, et al. Literacy promotion for Hispanic families in a primary care setting: a randomized, controlled trial. Pediatrics 1999;103:993–7.

[51] Mendelsohn AL, Mogilner LN, Dreyer BP, et al. The impact of a clinic-based literacy intervention on language development in inner-city preschool children. Pediatrics 2001;107: 130–4.

[52] Sharif I, Rieber S, Ozuah PO. Exposure to reach out and read and vocabulary outcomes in inner city preschoolers [erratum appears in J Natl Med Assoc 2002 sep;94(9):Following table of contents note: Reiber sarah [corrected to rieber sarah]]. J Natl Med Assoc 2002;94:171–7.

[53] Weitzman CC, Roy L, Walls T, et al. More evidence for reach out and read: a home-based study. Pediatrics 2004;113:1248–53.

[54] Lonigan CJ, Burgess SR, Anthony JL. Development of emergent literacy and early reading skills in preschool children: evidence from a latent-variable longitudinal study. Dev Psychol 2000;36:596–613.

[55] Administration for Children and Families (AFC), editor. Making a difference in the lives on infants and toddlers and their families: the impact of early Head Start. Washington, DC: Administration for Children and Families (AFC); 2002.

[56] Administration for Children, Youth and Families (ACYF), editor. Building their futures: how early Head Start programs are enhancing the lives of infants and toddlers in low-income families. Washington, DC: Administration for Children, Youth and Families (ACYF); 2001.

[57] Brooks-Gunn J, Klebanov PK, Liaw F, et al. Enhancing the development of low birthweight, premature infants: changes in cognition and behavior in the first three years. Child Dev 1993;64:736–53.

[58] Ramey CT, Campbell F. Children in poverty: child development and public policy. In: Huston A, editor. Poverty, early childhood education and academic competence: the Abecedarian experiment. New York: Cambridge University Press; 1991. p. 190–221.

[59] Espinosa L, Lesar S. Increasing language-minority family and child competencies for school success. Paper presented at the Annual Meeting of the American Educational Research Association, New Orleans, LA, April 4, 1994.

[60] Liontos LB. At-risk families and schools: becoming partners. Washington, DC: Office of Educational Research and Improvement 1992; RI88062004:170.

[61] National Center for Education Statistics. Family-child engagement in literacy activities: changes in participation between 1991 and 1993 (based on the National Household Education Survey: NCES 95-204 by DeeAnn Wright, Elvie Germino Hausken and Jerry West). Washington DC: US Department of Education; 1994.

[62] Espinosa LM. Hispanic parent involvement in early childhood programs. In: Clearinghouse on elementary and early childhood education. ED382412. ERIC Digest; 1995.

[63] Klass P, Needlman R, Zuckerman B. Reach out and read training manual. Boston: Reach Out and Read National Center; 1999.

PEDIATRIC CLINICS

OF NORTH AMERICA

ELSEVIER
SAUNDERS

Pediatr Clin N Am 54 (2007) 643–650

Index

Note: Page numbers of article titles are in **boldface** type.

A

Alphabetic principle, in reading, 507, 509–510

American Academy of Pediatrics, developmental screening algorithm of, 477

American Psychiatric Association
  autism spectrum disorder classification of, 469–470
  language disorder classification of, 439–441

Amplification, in hearing loss, 588–589

Anxiety disorders
  dyslexia with, 513
  language disorders with, 449, 458–459
  language impairment with, 534–535

Aphasia
  definition of, 594–595
  developmental. *See* Specific language impairment (mixed receptive-expressive language disorder).

Apraxia, 446–447
  case example of, 459–461
  in autism spectrum disorders, 472

Articulation disorders, 445–447

ASD. *See* Autism spectrum disorders.

Asperger's disorder
  description of, 470
  pragmatic language disorders in, 445
  social communication impairments in, 471
  speech disorders in, 475

Asymmetries, brain, 565–567

Attention-deficit/hyperactivity disorder
  dyslexia with, 512–513
  language disorders with, 449, 498, 500–501
  language impairment with, 533

Attentiveness, in pragmatic competence, 493

Auditory hypothesis
  of dyslexia, 547
  of language impairment, 548–549

Auditory processing abnormalities, 574–575

Auditory verbal processing deficits, 528–529

Auditory-temporal processing deficit, 453

Autism spectrum disorders, **469–481**
  brain abnormalities in, **563–583**
    asymmetry, 565–567
    auditory processing abnormalities, 574–575
    diencephalon, 567–568
    functional, 571–576
    macroanatomy of, 565–571
    motion perception abnormalities, 573
    neuropathology of, 576
    noise exclusion hypothesis of, 573–574
    sensory perception deficits, 571–572
    thalamic, 567–568
    volumetric differences, 568–571
  forms of, 469–470
  language disorders in, 470–471
    clinical implications of, 476–478
    in preschoolers, 471–474
    in toddlers, 471–474
    pragmatic, 445, 499
    prognosis for, 457–458
    recommendations for, 476–478
    regression, 429
    types of, 426–427
    versus normal school-aged children, 474–476
    versus normal toddlers, 471–474
  premature diagnosis of, 433
  screening for, 477
  social communication disorders in, 470–471

Moving?

Make sure your subscription moves with you!

To notify us of your new address, find your **Clinics Account Number** (located on your mailing label above your name), and contact customer service at:

E-mail: elspcs@elsevier.com

800-654-2452 (subscribers in the U.S. & Canada)
407-345-4000 (subscribers outside of the U.S. & Canada)

Fax number: 407-363-9661

Elsevier Periodicals Customer Service
6277 Sea Harbor Drive
Orlando, FL 32887-4800

*To ensure uninterrupted delivery of your subscription, please notify us at least 4 weeks in advance of move.